HEALTH PROMOTION AND WELLNESS
An Evidence-Based Guide to
Clinical Preventive Services

HEALTH PROMOTION AND WELLNESS

An Evidence-Based Guide to Clinical Preventive Services

EDITORS

Cheryl Hawk, DC, PhD, CHES

Professor and Director of Clinical Research
Logan College of Chiropractic/University Programs
Chesterfield, Missouri

Will Evans, DC, PhD, MCHES

Professor and Dean of Academic Affairs
United States Sports Academy
Daphne, Alabama

Wolters Kluwer | Lippincott Williams & Wilkins
Health
Philadelphia • Baltimore • New York • London
Buenos Aires • Hong Kong • Sydney • Tokyo

Acquisitions Editor: Brian Brown
Senior Product Manager: Dave Murphy
Senior Manufacturing Manager: Benjamin Rivera
Marketing Manager: Lisa Lawrence
Design Coordinator: Doug Smock
Production Service: S4Carlisle Publishing Services

Printed in China

Library of Congress Cataloging-in-Publication Data
Health promotion and wellness : an evidence-based guide to clinical preventive services / editors, Cheryl Hawk, Will Evans.
    p. ; cm.
Includes bibliographical references.
ISBN 978-1-4511-2023-3
ISBN 1-4511-2023-0
I. Hawk, Cheryl. II. Evans, Will, 1961-
[DNLM: 1. Health Promotion—methods. 2. Complementary Therapies. 3. Counseling. 4. Health Behavior. 5. Preventive Health Services. WA 590]
    362.1—dc23
                                                                    2012034645

Care has been taken to confirm the accuracy of the information presented and to describe generally accepted practices. However, the authors, editors, and publisher are not responsible for errors or omissions or for any consequences from application of the information in this book and make no warranty, expressed or implied, with respect to the currency, completeness, or accuracy of the contents of the publication. Application of the information in a particular situation remains the professional responsibility of the practitioner.

The authors, editors, and publisher have exerted every effort to ensure that drug selection and dosage set forth in this text are in accordance with current recommendations and practice at the time of publication. However, in view of ongoing research, changes in government regulations, and the constant flow of information relating to drug therapy and drug reactions, the reader is urged to check the package insert for each drug for any change in indications and dosage and for added warnings and precautions. This is particularly important when the recommended agent is a new or infrequently employed drug.

Some drugs and medical devices presented in the publication have Food and Drug Administration (FDA) clearance for limited use in restricted research settings. It is the responsibility of the health care provider to ascertain the FDA status of each drug or device planned for use in their clinical practice.

To purchase additional copies of this book, call our customer service department at (800) 638-3030 or fax orders to (301) 223-2320. International customers should call (301) 223-2300.

Visit Lippincott Williams & Wilkins on the Internet: at LWW.com. Lippincott Williams & Wilkins customer service representatives are available from 8:30 am to 6 pm, EST.

10 9 8 7 6 5 4 3 2 1

CONTENTS

ACKNOWLEDGMENTS

The authors would like to thank Cathy Evans for encouraging us to write this book, and without whom it would not have been possible.

CONTRIBUTING AUTHORS

Karen E. Bülow, MLS, AHIP
Assistant Professor
Texas Chiropractic College
Pasadena, Texas

Mike Perko, PhD, MCHES, FAAHE
Associate Professor
Department of Public Health Education
School of Health and Human Sciences
University of North Carolina
Greensboro, North Carolina

Daniel Redwood, DC
Professor
Cleveland Chiropractic College – Kansas City
Overland Park, Kansas

Ronald D. Williams, Jr., PhD, CHES
Assistant Professor
Department of Food Science, Nutrition, & Health
    Promotion
Mississippi State University
Starkville, Mississippi

HEALTH PROMOTION AND WELLNESS
An Evidence-Based Guide to
Clinical Preventive Services

CHAPTER 1

Introduction

Cheryl Hawk and Marion W. Evans, Jr.

Disease prevention and health promotion have become increasingly important as health care costs in the United States continue to spiral out of control. In 2007, US health care expenditures reached US $2.4 trillion, 17% of the gross domestic product. Health care outcomes have not kept pace with expenditures. The United States currently spends the most on health care while having the lowest-ranked health care outcomes of all developed countries.[1] One factor contributing to this situation is that our system is built on a fee-for-service model of treating disease, with disease prevention being more of an "add-on" than a central feature, and health promotion and wellness an afterthought, at best. The new Patient Protection and Affordable Care Act (PPACA) is designed to address this issue, requiring Medicare and commercial health plans to pay for preventive services graded A and B by the U.S. Preventive Services Task Force (USPSTF), with no out-of-pocket cost to consumers. For this new direction to be successful, it is imperative that health care providers, whether conventional or complementary and alternative medicine (CAM), are appropriately trained and equipped to address the need for preventive care.

At the time we are writing this introduction, news has broken suggesting that the rate of type 2 diabetes, related to lifestyle choices in most adults, has doubled since 1980 and will double again within the next ten years.[2] Physical inactivity, poor diet, and excessive use of alcohol and tobacco still remain the four most significant threats related to the choices Americans make that will shorten their lives. Table 1.1 summarizes the leading "actual" causes of death—the lifestyle related factors that contribute to mortality.[3] For many, the morbidity and disability that will precede years of life lost will place limitations on their ability to work, play with grandchildren, and do the things they love. Figure 1.1 shows the leading causes of disability for U.S. adults in 2005.

Because of the importance of chronic lifestyle-related diseases, the World Health Organization (WHO) now recommends that preventive health care become integrated into the fabric of the health care encounter, which would represent a global paradigm shift.[4] WHO states that the following components are essential to accomplish this integration:

Emphasize integrated, preventive health care.
Implement policies strengthening preventive and health promotion services.
Institute patient information systems that support patients' self-efficacy in improving their health behavior.
Make prevention part of every health care encounter.

It has been known for many years that health care providers are among the most powerful people to cue others to take action related to health or healthier behaviors.[5] To leverage this in our society, we need every health care provider to advise and provide resources for patients to make positive changes in their health. Yet when asked why they do not promote health and advise patients more frequently, providers often state that they do not have the time; that they cannot get paid for these services; and that they feel patients are not going to be receptive. However, these perceptions are not entirely true. For example, the new PPACA requires that insurance cover all preventive services with a USPSTF rating of A or B.[6,7] Furthermore, there are preventive services billing codes already in existence, which many practitioners are not aware of, or do not think are reimbursable. Finally, many studies indicate that patients would like greater opportunities to partner with their clinicians to explore ways to get and stay well.

TABLE 1.1	Actual Causes of Death in the United States, 2000
Causes of Death	**Percentage**
Tobacco use	18
Poor diet and physical inactivity	17
Alcohol	4
Microbial agents	3
Toxic agents	2
Motor vehicle	2
Firearms	1
Sexual behavior	1
Illegal drug use	<1

Source: Mokdad et al., Actual Causes of Death in the United States, 2000. *JAMA*. 2004;291(10):1238-1245.

PURPOSE OF THIS BOOK

This book is geared for health care providers, particularly CAM clinicians. CAM practitioners, of which doctors of chiropractic (DCs) are the most commonly used type,[8] have not yet been integrated into national efforts to provide all Americans with much-needed prevention and health promotion services. However, CAM continues to grow in popularity, with about 24% of American adults using CAM providers in 2007,[9]

and it is important that this branch of health care become as well-versed in prevention and health promotion approaches as conventional practitioners. Since CAM is usually used to supplement, rather than substitute for, conventional health care, CAM and conventional providers might collaborate to reinforce their comanaged patients' health messages—particularly since CAM users tend to be more interested in improving their health behavior than nonusers.[10] CAM practice is also a good setting for health promotion and prevention counseling, since research suggests that the increased energy resulting from CAM therapies can be helpful to patients in making health behavior changes.[11]

This book is organized into two sections. The first section gives information on risks, ways providers can assess for risk, and tools they can use to advise and help patients move forward. The second section is a tool kit with information, resources, tools, and other items that can help the clinician provide evidence-based, patient-centered information to their patients.

In this book, we have focused on the most common risk factors that are also amenable to provider-based counseling. For instance, clean water and air are critical for survival and good health, but these are public health issues best addressed by laws and social change. This book addresses personal health issues related to individual risks because these are the ones clinicians can most successfully address with patients. Therefore, we do not attempt

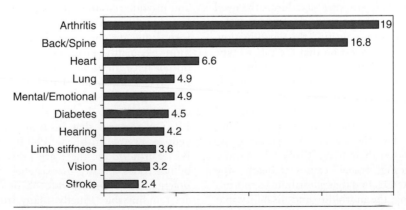

Figure 1.1. Top 10 causes of disability in U.S. adults. Bars show percentage of adult population reporting eac condition to be the main cause of their self-reported disability.

Source: Centers for Disease Control and Prevention. Older, more diverse population and longer lifespans contributing to increase in deabetes 2010. www.cdc.gov/media/pressrel/2010/r101022.html.

to address every "macro" level public health risk, or even every health risk in every patient. Another area we do not address is treatment. Although we acknowledge that patients most often seek clinical care to receive appropriate treatment, our focus is on screening patients for risks and reducing those risks where this is possible. Sometimes we may be able to intervene at the level of primary prevention, sometimes secondary, and sometimes only at the tertiary level. Our purpose in this book is to provide the screening, prevention, health promotion, and advising information and resources that will complement your routine care of the patients you serve.

How to Use This Book

As is the case with most textbooks, this one will become outdated as new information and evidence appear. Although many of the risk factors we address in this book will still be prevalent decades from now, new and better ways of assisting patients to modify them will arise as research continues. This means that lifelong learning is a necessity for all clinicians. Use this book as an introduction to the topics we present, but keep abreast of changes that are occurring in the identification of risks, methods of treatment, preventive efforts, and new tools that will always surface that can help a patient be successful in adoption of a healthier lifestyle. This book is not intended to be the end-all or even to address everything that clinicians might wish to do to promote health and wellness in their practices. Rather, we intend to provide readers with the basic elements necessary to help their patients change their health behavior related to the most prevalent risk factors, and to serve as a springboard to keep pace with the latest evidence arising in the applied science of wellness, prevention, and health promotion.

Literature Cited

1. Muennig PA, Glied SA. What changes in survival rates tell us about US health care. *Health Aff (Millwood)*. 2010;29(11):2105–2113.
2. Centers for Disease Control and Prevention. Older, more diverse population and longer lifespans contributing to increase in diabetes, 2010. www.cdc.gov/media/pressrel/2010/r101022.html.
3. Mokdad AH, Marks JS, Stroup DF, Gerberding JL. Actual Causes of Death in the United States, 2000. *JAMA*. 2004;291(10):1238-1245.
4. World Health Organization. Integrating prevention into health care. WHO *Fact sheet No. 172 revised October* 2002; *Indian J Med Sci*. 2002; 56(12):619–621.
5. Rosenstock IM, Strecher VJ, Becker MH. Social learning theory and the Health Belief Model. *Health Educ Q*. 1988;15(2):175–183.
6. Koh HK, Sebelius KG. Promoting prevention through the Affordable Care Act. *N Engl J Med*. 2010;363(14):1296–1299.
7. USPSTF. *Guide to Clinical Preventive Services*. Washington, DC: Agency for Healthcare Research and Quality (AHRQ); 2010.
8. Barnes PM, Powell-Griner E, McFann K, et al. Complementary and alternative medicine use among adults: United States, 2002. *Adv Data*. 2004;343:1–19.
9. Barnes PM, Bloom B, Nahin RL. Complementary and alternative medicine use among adults and children: United States, 2007. *Natl Health Stat Report*. 2008;12:1–23.
10. National Center for Complementary and Alternative Medicine. *Draft Strategic Plan*. Bethesda, MD: National Institutues of Health; 2010.
11. Williams-Piehota P, Sirois FM, Bann CM, et al.. Agents of change: how do complementary and alternative medicine providers play a role in health behavior change? *Altern Ther Health Med*. 2011;17(1):22–30.

CHAPTER 2

Understanding Health Behavior

Marion W. Evans, Jr.

INTRODUCTION

Behavior is among the most important factors contributing to premature morbidity and mortality, with the decisions of tobacco use, physical inactivity, and choices made regarding diet being among the most likely contributors to poor health.[1] Patients have the ability to choose differently in each of the areas, so why do people still smoke, refuse to get regular physical activity, and eat a diet putting them on direct course for pathology? Perhaps a better understanding of the complexities of this subject can be gained from a knowledge of health behavior and how people change, or fail to in many cases. The focus of this chapter is to introduce the reader to concepts used in public health education and health behavior, and to emphasize how they can be applied in clinical practice to help patients increase their success for change.

If you were to wake up tomorrow and decide you were going to become a cigarette smoker, go down to the local quick stop and buy a pack of cigarettes, you would find a label placed on the side of the pack that essentially says smoking causes cancer and may kill you. So why would anyone actually go through with the purchase? Americans do so at a prevalence of about 20%,[2] even though the first US Surgeon General report[3] on the dangers of tobacco use was publicized in 1964 and the dangers continue to appear in the news regularly. So relative to smoking there must be other factors at work. Otherwise, no one in their right mind would smoke.

Although a quick look at any table or chart on the causes of death listed by their diagnoses will show heart disease, stroke, cancer, and other diseases at the top of the list, when it comes to actual causes of death (Fig. 2.1), we see these major modifiable behaviors surfacing as the true causes of early morbidity and mortality. Even the

Healthy People Initiatives[4] lists priority areas that deal mostly with behaviors that can be changed simply through the will of the potentially affected population (Table 2.1).

Chronic diseases that take years to develop are typically caused by years of poor choices. However, even in the case of infectious diseases, there is usually a behavioral component involved. Think about West Nile virus (WNV) or human immunodeficiency virus (HIV), which causes acquired immunodeficiency syndrome (AIDS); each of those viral diseases has behavioral components. Those who choose to go outside at dusk and dawn in the summer months with no insect repellent risk a mosquito bite that carries the WNV and a potential increase in risk of infection. And of course everyone knows about unprotected sex and the HIV risks this carries, but still new cases of HIV are noted every year.

THE ROLE OF BEHAVIOR IN THE CAUSE OF DISEASE

Behavior is shaped at an early age in most cultures. Depending on what part of the country or world one is born in, there may be factors that are seen early on as being beyond the control of the individual. For example, if you were born in the rural south, you may eat fried pickles or have cornbread at every meal. Sweet tea with a lot of added sugar is considered a delicacy in the south. If you are taught by your family that these are the foods native to your social culture then you are more likely to grow up eating a certain way. Today, you can even purchase fried Twinkies and fried Coke at the Texas State Fair! Other cultures have habituated certain practices or diets that may predispose the population to increased or decreased risk for disease. Even religious groups have nuances to their diets that may alter health

Tobacco use
Poor diet and inactivity
Alcohol use
Microbes
Toxins
Motor vehicle accidents
Firearms
Risky sexual behaviors
Illicit drug use

Figure 2.1. Actual causes of death.
Source: From Mokdad AH, Marks JS, Stroup DF, et al. Actual causes of death in the United States, 2000. *JAMA*. 2004;291(1):1238–1245, with permission.

TABLE 2.1	Leading Health Indicators from *Healthy People 2010*
Physical activity	
Overweight and obesity	
Tobacco use	
Substance abuse	
Responsible sexual behavior	
Mental health	
Injury and violence	
Environmental quality	
Immunization	
Access to health care	

risks, one way or another. Some do not advocate the use of caffeine, red meat, pork, or other specific foods. Seventh Day Adventists, for example, promote a diet high in fruits, vegetables, and nuts that is also low in red and other meats. These choices, based on religious predilection may affect the health of those who adhere to them.

Many behaviors are indeed shaped early in life and can be difficult to change. Anyone who has made an attempt to change a behavior personally can attest to this fact. In some cases, we just don't want to change. Some behaviors that have negative consequences are pleasurable to us. Sweet tea tastes good! The concept of behavior as an antecedent to health has been studied for many years and will probably be studied for many more. From this research, health scientists have developed health behavioral theories, many of which predict individual behaviors or account for social/cultural influences that in some way shape the choices we make. Therefore, health behavioral theories are models that have been tested and essentially provide logical frameworks that can predict how people behave. Placed appropriately in the planning process, they can be used to try and assist people in making better, healthy choices and can assist the health care provider in identifying points to motivate the patient to start the process of change. They may also assist communities in planning or organizing health events or in shaping cultural norms toward a healthier lifestyle.

Micro features are factors within the control or inherent position of individuals. They may include knowledge, attitudes, beliefs, medical history, genetic predisposition, and even family history of disease. Macro factors involve the larger socioecological issues that could predispose one to premature morbidity and mortality or not. These may be the neighborhood a person lives in, the physical environmental issues around them, or social/peer influences and perhaps policies at work or laws within the state they reside in. Taking in to account a variety of micro and macro factors in a population can enhance behavior change associated with health choices.

HEALTH BEHAVIOR THEORY

Health behavioral theories generally fall into two categories: explanatory theories and planning theories.[5] Explanatory theories look at the behaviors of individuals and how they may be influenced by factors inherent to the individual, such as knowledge, attitudes, or beliefs, and in many cases how the outside environment influences people. In this case, ecological/environmental factors include not only the physical environment one may be living in but also socioenvironmental issues or problems that facilitate poor or healthy decisions or habits. Planning theories tend to focus on how those in public health can best plan large-scale or community-wide interventions so that the designated message reaches the right people in a way that gets their attention.[6] Each of these categories may be used to frame research efforts or to better understand how populations may behave in certain circumstances as well.

Explanatory Theories

THE ECOLOGICAL THEORY OF HEALTH BEHAVIOR

The ecological theory of health promotion was developed by McLeroy and colleagues[7] and has five basic constructs that make up the model. These include intrapersonal factors, interpersonal factors, community norms, institutional policies, and public policy or laws. Intrapersonal issues are those inherent to the individual. These may include knowledge, attitudes, beliefs held by the individual, together with unchangeable factors such as genetics or their past medical history, which at some point cannot be altered. Interpersonal issues surround the relationships that an individual has with significant others. At times, peer groups, family members, coworkers, and even the family doctor could have either a positive or a negative influence on the choices an individual makes. Community norms can be another factor inherent to the decision-making process. As stated above, we are shaped by the cultures we grew up in or live in and they can have positive or negative effects. What is accepted by a community can vary from place to place, and this is known to have an effect on health. Policies can be made at the local level or even at the institutional level. The recent issue of cola machines in schools is one such issue that has influenced kids in a negative way, and along with the decision to reduce the number of physical education hours in school may have assisted in increasing risks for adolescent obesity.

Laws are also factors that can affect health. Recent changes in laws on where one can smoke, seat-belt use, cell phone use, and motorcycle helmet use are all examples of how a change in the law can bring about changes in population health status or risk levels. Figure 2.2 summarizes a report from the Institute of Medicine on the cardiovascular effects of secondhand cigarette smoke, and how laws restricting smoking have altered risks.[8] The ecological model frames a logical explanation for how not only individual actions affect health but how social phenomena can play a significant role in how we make choices or how a population behaves. Therefore, it is not responsible of health care providers to simply state that the individual needs to make better choices. While this may be true, the issue is typically much more complex than simply getting a patient or a group of people to choose a different behavioral pattern. The social circumstances will often be too overwhelming for an individual to make the right choice, and for that reason social factors must always be taken into account when we want to help people make positive changes in their behavior. Table 2.2 provides an example of how health care providers may apply efforts to help their community change health behaviors.

THE HEALTH BELIEF MODEL

The health belief model (HBM) is one of the oldest explanatory models of health behavior.[9] Developed by the U.S. Public Health Service in the 1950s, scientists wanted to know why individuals would not come in for a free screening to determine their risks of tuberculosis (TB). What they discovered indicated that perceptions are indeed everything. The constructs of the HBM are based on how people perceive risks and how they act on those perceptions. First, perceived susceptibility is a major factor. The researchers found that if a person did not feel they were susceptible for TB, for example, whether they were

---

A 2009 Institute of Medicine report concluded that second hand smoke exposure increases one's risks of heart disease by 25%–30%. The report also found that even low levels of exposure in animal experiments cause possible harm to the cardiovascular system. The review included 11 studies that also show when smoking bans go into effect in various areas heart attacks go down. All of the studies demonstrated reduction in the number of heart attacks with decreases ranging from 6%–47%.

In this example of how policy could reduce health risks, the Institute of Medicine concluded that smoking bans can, "have a substantial impact on public health... as well as save lives."

Figure 2.2. Second-hand smoke exposure and heart disease—How public policy can reduce health risks.
Source: From Institute of Medicine of the National Academies, Brief Report, October 2009. *Secondhand Smoke Exposure and Cardiovascular Effects: Making Sense of the Evidence,* with permission.

TABLE 2.2	Ecological Model of How a Health Care Provider Can Influence Health and Health Policy
Intrapersonal issues	Help patients and community with increased knowledge, change attitudes and beliefs, and enhance self-efficacy and skill-set
Interpersonal issues	Help identify support within the family, teach patient to prepare for behavior change, and provide resources or referral to specialists, coaches, or counselors
(Community) Institutional issues	Lobby for institutional changes in schools, local, state, or national agencies, promote national standards, and express goals such as Healthy People initiatives
(Community) Norms	Support local groups initiating change, encourage walking paths, bike paths, safety, and community health initiatives aimed at groups and communities
(Community) Public policy	Lobby for better smoking ordinances, helmet laws, and support existing policies and public health programs that enhance health

or not, they would not come in for the screening. Next, they found the persons needed to feel they were at risk of something they perceived to be significant. Perceived significance meant that they perceived a threat that was not only real, but could cause a significant health problem for them personally. Note that it is "perception" driving behavior and may have nothing to do with reality. Perceived benefits of taking action are the next construct in the model. What kind of benefit does taking action have? Is this benefit significant for the one taking action? What will taking action bring? To some, it could bring bad news, which may factor into the decision-making process. Therefore, what are perceived barriers to taking action? If a person does not want bad news, that is a barrier. Costs and time out of a busy schedule are also factors that tend to be perceived as barriers by patients and individuals. The health care provider needs to take into account each of these to get a person to take action according to the model.

Two added factors to the model have been put in place since the inception of the HBM. Self-efficacy, a component of other theories, means, does a person feel they have the ability to take the needed action that perhaps they are being told or asked to take? Cue to action is the last component. In other words, how can a person be encouraged to take action? Who or what can cue them to act? In many cases, it is felt that the health care provider is the most powerful cue to get a person to take action about their health. Typically, the

HBM is used to look at how to get individuals to take a single action such as come in for a flu shot or some other action that is a onetime act or at least once every so often. However, health care providers need to realize that the individual may regard their advice as the most important when compared with family, friends, and other significant people in their lives. We should not fail to advise our patients when we have the opportunity for this specific reason. Celebrities, friends, family members, and others can cue people to take action, but people look to their providers to advise them on what to do when health is the issue. This does not mean they will take action or be successful when they do, but this needed action must be known in order to be taken for a chance at successful behavior change. Advising small, attainable goals is another way to enhance the process as this will also build self-efficacy with patients. Providers should also have resources for patients so that if they choose action they are not let down by not knowing what to do next. Additional sections of the text will address developing resources for patients and how to facilitate behavior change as a step at a time.

TRANSTHEORETICAL MODEL (STAGES OF CHANGE)

Psychologists developed the transtheoretical model, known commonly as the "stages model."[10] Stages of Change are stages of susceptibility a person goes through in relation to their willingness or interest in making a behavior change. Originally developed to better explain how those with addictions behave, Stages of Change has five constructs. Although people fall into one of the stages, they may not move through them in a linear manner. That is, they may move back and forth within the model prior to successful modification of a health behavior.

The first stage is precontemplation. In this stage, a person has no interest in making a behavioral change and in fact, may not be aware they have a need to change anything. We can use physical activity as an example. A precontemplator has no intention of exercising or increasing physical activity levels within the next 6 months. If advised by the health care provider, they may state they don't like to exercise or that they just don't have the time. A signal is then sent that says, "I'm not interested."

A contemplator then is one who has an interest in making a change but has not done anything to facilitate that at the current time. They have plans to make a change within the next 6 months. Perhaps in late November, they decide they need to lose weight and set a New Year's resolution to increase physical activity levels and join the YMCA. They have not acted but they have plans. Preparation is next. In December, they visit the Y and inquire about costs, programs, and how to get started. In the action stage they have taken some action. They have been to the Y for the first time, joined an aerobics or spinning class, and started the process of change. In the maintenance stage, they have maintained the new behavior (regular physical activity) for at least 6 months.

It is important to note that with patients in particular, one should respect the stage the person is in, and work with them to move them through the stages. Trying to force a change into the life of a precontemplator will only frustrate the doctor and the patient. A premise of all explanatory theories is that people value their health. In cases of addiction and among adolescents, the models sometimes run into difficulty as adolescents may feel invincible to poor health or death, and those with drug addictions may not have a clear perception of anything, much less a desire to change behavior toward healthy actions. The health care provider should be aware of this should they encounter these subsets of the population in practice and be prepared to make the appropriate referral to another specialist when this is clinically indicated. The goal of the provider should be to assist the patient in moving toward positive change. A brochure to the current smoker who is a precontemplator, for example, may say, "Not interested in quitting—at least think about it," while one aimed at those in the contemplation stage or preparation stage may show the patient simple things to do to start the action process.[11]

In the process of behavior change we have already stated that a minority of patients is told by their doctors to change an unhealthy behavior often only after a disease process is in place or a threat is imminent. In addition, an even smaller number are given information on how to successfully make a change. Having stage-based resources in place and knowing how hard to encourage the patient can be very important in increasing the number of patients who make successful attempts at behavior change. This will also reduce burnout of the provider who may often think no one wants to hear their positive behavioral messaging, when in reality, there may be plenty. Encouraging those who are successful is also very important as there may not be others in that patient's life doing so. A pat on the back when appropriate or stating how proud you are of them for their success cannot be overstated. This may be all they need to reinforce a needed but not so positive change at home. This can be especially so when a spouse shares similar risks and doesn't want to change personal health habits.

SOCIAL COGNITIVE THEORY

Developed by Bandura in the mid-1980s, social cognitive theory (SCT) suggests that personal factors, the environment, and behavior are interrelated and each has an effect on the other.[12] This "reciprocal determinism" is a key factor within the theory. Behavior change can occur if a person feels they have the self-efficacy to make the needed changes, set reasonable goals, and have expectations related to potential outcomes of the behavior change that they consider favorable. Other points considered by the theory are behavioral capability, expectations, observational learning, and reinforcements. Those are described in more detail in Table 2.3.

Planning and Communication Theories

There are numerous planning theories available for use at the community level, and some can have constructs that are of use for planning health care interventions as well. Communications theories

TABLE 2.3	Potential Use of Social Cognitive Theory in Practice Setting	
Behavioral capability	Knowledge and skills needed to make behavior change	A lapel button is a button or insignia that is pinned to a doctors' lab coat (on the lapel) and are common to various health education campaigns. This was an "intern" lapel button used on intern lab coats.
Expectations	What the patients anticipate as the outcomes of the changes they will make	Accentuate the positive, gain-frame messages to state what these changes will bring rather than the negatives of not changing; stress lifelong change versus a quick fix
Reinforcements	Positive or negative reinforcements that may keep patients on track or throw them off	Encourage, reward positive changes

are specific to how to get a message across to an audience and may have value for practitioners in learning how patients receive messages to change behavior. Although an in-depth discussion is beyond the scope of the chapter, a few are discussed here. First, the PRECEDE–PROCEED planning model developed by Green and Kreuter is considered an extensive planning model for various community health promotion programs.[13] The theory uses a variety of assessment tools to look at the risks to a group or community and then takes into account various strategies to make an intervention or education campaign more successful, and last, adds an evaluation algorithm to the end. The model looks at risks to the individual caused by both the individual's actions and the environmental features that may be at work as well.[6]

The PRECEDE part of the acronym stands for "Predisposing, Reinforcing, Enabling Constructs in Educational/Environmental Diagnosis and Evaluation." This prompts one to look at those factors that are making the existing behavior possible and the issues related to the social environment one is in, in addition to the educational needs that may be apparent. In a sense, the situation is diagnosed in this part of the model. The PROCEED component stands for "Policy, Regulatory, and Organizational Constructs in Educational and Environmental Development." Added later, this part of the model allows interpretation of the information from the PRECEDE part and moves one toward the actual implementation of a program and then evaluation. A summary of the phases of the model and their applications can be seen in Table 2.4. Of particular importance to anyone trying to assist

patients with a behavioral change are those predisposing, enabling, and reinforcing factors that are a part of this model. Knowing what may predispose or enable a person to change to a healthier behavior or at least prompt one to consider a change can be critical to assisting them. Reinforcement of the new behavior is also very important. If the health care provider is the only one prompting the change and monitoring the patient's progress, reinforcement of the new behavior is a need that cannot be overstated. Communications theories and methods will be discussed in a later chapter 4 of the text, but some tools to start the dialogue related to behavior change are certainly appropriate here.

Assisting Patients in the Process of Behavior Change

SMALL STEPS

Earlier, the concept of self-efficacy was introduced. This is the perception that one has the ability or skills to make a change that is requested of them or needed. Building this self-efficacy is as important as teaching actual skills needed for behavior change. For example, a person may know they need to increase physical activity but if they don't think they have the time or money required to go to a gym, they will feel they can't be successful and may not even make an attempt at change. Providing short messages about simple things a person can do to increase levels of activity may build that self-efficacy when they see it is not as complex as they once thought, it takes less time, and the effects of physical activity are

TABLE 2.4	Summary of PRECEDE–PROCEED Applications
Phase 1: Social Assessment or Diagnosis	Looks at the broad, social picture in a community
Phase 2: Epidemiological Assessment	Starts the planning process with the known epidemiological situation in a community and identifies key health issues and who is at risk
Phase 3: Behavioral and Environmental Assessment	The behaviors that put the community at risk, environmental issues—external and/or physical
Phase 4: Educational and Ecological Assessment	Identify educational needs, social norms, socioecological issues that need to be addressed
Phase 5: Administrative and Policy Assessment	Key policies or administrative issues that increase risks
Phase 6: Implementation	The plan is implemented on the basis of the assessments above
Phase 7: Evaluation	*Process*—Is it working, and what are problems that need to be corrected
Phase 8: Evaluation	*Impact*—Is there evidence of short-term gains from the program
Phase 9: Evaluation	*Outcome*—Did the program change health outcomes or have positive, long-term effects

accumulated over the course of the week. Perhaps they can

• park further from the store when they shop;
• walk their dog for 10 minutes a day;
• take the stairs rather than an elevator;
• exercise between commercials on television;
• walk the parking lot perimeter at work during their lunch or 15-minute break.

The main idea is to set small, achievable goals that a patient can attain to build the needed self-efficacy, and with added confidence, more behavioral change can occur. The Centers for Disease Control and Prevention (CDC) and the U.S. Department of Health and Human Services state that 150 minutes of physical activity per week is essential.[14] Helping patients find ways to accumulate this takes a creative scheme and understanding of where that patient is in the stages of change.

MESSAGE FRAMING

Message framing is a part of a field called health communications. In message framing typically, one seeks to get a message to break through all of the other messages or noise a person has to deal with each day. For most people who have needed to change a behavior for some time, they have likely heard a message that they need to make a change. "Lose 30 pounds before I see you again. . ." or "You really shouldn't smoke. . ." are messages many people have heard before. So what can one do to get the message through to the patients so they take action? First, the message will probably work better if gain-framed. Gain-framing essentially means we emphasize what a person will gain from making a needed change in opposition to a loss-frame message that indicates what they will lose if they fail to change.[15] Although negative framing or fear appeals are used (e.g., "This is your brain on drugs. . ."), if we accentuate the positive, we keep the patient focused on what the new behavior will bring and that tends to be better in the long run. However, if a serious risk remains, it is essential to balance the gain-frame messaging with actual risks of not making a change.[16]

Starting the process of advising patients about needed changes can be intimidating if this has not been an area where one has traditionally felt comfortable or, in some cases, responsible for practicing. However, as has been stated, many patients never hear a message to change or never received the tools to be effective. The ABC's of health promotion[17] may help along with the Surgeon General's 5 A's. [18] The 5 A's deal with ways to remember the steps in moving a patient from being unaware that they need to change all the way to follow-up to see how they are progressing. The first 'A' is "Ask" about the risk behavior. "Do you smoke?" (This can be done on intake paperwork if needed.) If they do, "Advise" them they need to make a quit attempt. "Assess" their willingness to do so, and "Assist" them with this process if they want to make a change. And last, "Arrange for follow-up." The worst thing that can be done is to advise but not offer assistance and resources and fail to follow-up. Also, keep in mind the 5 A's can be used for any behavior change idea. They have been used mostly frequently for smoking cessation advising but apply them at will!

The ABC's of Health Promotion

The ABC's of health promotion[17] allow us to aim at patients with whom we have already established a good relationship. Many practitioners may feel uncomfortable at first when it comes to taking on the role of cueing patients to take action. For this reason it makes sense to start with those patients who are regular users of your services. The ABC's serve as a reminder of the very basics of where to start:

- **A**—*Assess* your patient for their needs regarding helpful behavior changes.
- **B**—Extol the *Benefits* of the behavior change rather than the negatives of continued current behaviors.
- **C**—Use *Clinical* preventive care or check-up visits as the jumping-off point toward making this a part of your routine.
- **S**—Provide *Stay-the-Course Messages* when patients seem to be having a tough go at behavior changes. This will encourage them to keep trying at a time when the doctor may be their only ally.

As the issue of advising each patient becomes more and more comfortable, you can start the process of advising newer patients earlier in their care. This will give additional opportunities over the course of treatment to engage them and, therefore, add to a potential dose response on messaging. The more messages a patient receives, the more opportunities they have to make

a change. Don't give up. Keep advising and be sure to give every patient the opportunity for a needed behavior change, and provide them with the appropriate resources to be successful; not just those who are overweight, smoke, or look like they need it. Reducing a risk before they develop a health problem should be the goal.

SUMMARY

Getting comfortable with the role of cueing patients to change negative health behaviors takes time and practice. The good news is you are among the most credible, powerful people to cue them as a health care provider. Studies show that when advised to make a behavioral change by a physician or chiropractor, more than 80% of patients state they made an attempt at that behavior change and, in addition, are more likely to share that information with others.[19,20]

Here are some key things to remember:

- Use a clear, strong message as the doctor— "As your doctor I believe this is one of the most important things you can do."
- Remember to "gain-frame" the message to accentuate the positive.
- Start with those patients who feel comfortable with you and you with them, such as the regular maintenance care patient—Use your ABC's.
- Start to build a set of resources for patients so they may be successful if they choose to attempt change (brochures, CDC downloads, websites, lists of local programs, or partners).
- Encourage and reward them often.

Assisting the patient with behavior changes can be very rewarding. Some patients may apply changes suggested by a clinician that they never imagined could work or help them. When they do it successfully, it unleashes a powerful process that moves them toward greater self-efficacy and control of their personal health, perhaps in a way they have never experienced, and both patient and doctor will recall a positive experience once that happens. Table 2.5 summarizes how theory is used to design a smoking cessation education campaign to increase intern engagement of patients[21] using the 5 A's and part of the PRECEDE–PROCEDE constructs.

TABLE 2.5	Matrix with Predisposing, Enabling, and Reinforcing Constructs and Use of 5 A's for Smoking Cessation Advising by Interns		
5 A's	**Predisposing**	**Enabling**	**Reinforcing**
Ask patient about smoking status	Have box stamped on patient chart to remind and allow intern to check off tasks from asking to arranging follow-up.	Teach 5 A's to interns and allow opportunity to practice advising roles, cover tobacco use in intake paperwork, review of systems on all patients	Have staff doctors model this advising role, require intern to review smoking status on every patient and in clinic entrance examination assessments
	Intern lapel button on smoke-free campaign	Intern lapel button	Intern lapel button
Advise patient to quit	Printed 5 A's pocket card for intern to carry in pocket to remind them what to say	Have stage-based brochures on file and easy to access for patients and interns	In-service and how and when to use each brochure or literature
Assess willingness to quit	Use of check box on chart, cover in report of findings with patients stresses need to quit and link to chronic spine disease	Teach advising and assessment skills to interns and allow opportunity to practice advising roles	Have staff doctors model advising role, assess on clinic entrance
Assist patient	Have stage-based brochures and literature and list of free smoking cessation programs in area available to give patient	Offer to partner with family doctor to get needed medications or assess use of nicotine replacement therapy	Remind patient periodically of need to quit and that intern is willing to assist when ready, chart discussion threads in chart
Arrange for follow-up	Use check boxes on chart to note the progress of the patient and set follow-up date in chart	Put post-it on outside of chart to remind the intern to follow up	Follow up with patient as scheduled

Literature Cited

1. Mokdad, AH, Marks JS, Stroup DF, et al. Actual causes of death in the United States, 2000. *JAMA.* 2004;291(10):1238–1245. doi:10.1001/jama.291.10.1238.
2. Centers for Disease Control and Prevention. Adult cigarette smoking in the United States: current estimate, 2009. http://www.cdc.gov/tobacco/data_statistics/fact_sheets/adult_data/cig_smoking/index.htm. Accessed February 17, 2010.
3. The Reports of the Surgeon General. *The 1964 Report on Smoking and Health.* http://profiles.nlm.nih.gov/NN/Views/Exhibit/narrative/smoking.html. Accessed February 17, 2010.
4. Healthy People Initiative. http://www.healthy-people.gov. Accessed February 17, 2010.
5. Glanz K, Rimer BK. *Theory at a Glance: a Guide for Health Promotion Practice.* Bethesda, MD: National Cancer Institute; 2005. Publication No. 05-3896.
6. Glanz K, Rimer BK, Viswanath K. Eds. *Health Behavior and Health Education: Theory, Research and Practice.* 4th ed. San Francisco, CA; Jossey-Bass; 2008:23–40.
7. McLeroy KR, Bibeau D, Steckler A, et al. An ecological perspective on health promotion programs. *Health Educ Q.* 1988;15(4):351–377.
8. Institute of Medicine. *Secondhand Smoke Exposure and Cardiovascular Effects: Making Sense of the Evidence.* Washington, DC: Institute of Medicine of The National Academies.

http://www.iom.edu/secondhandsmokecveffects. Accessed February 25, 2010.

9. Rosenstock IM, Strecher VJ, Becker MH. Social learning theory and the Health Belief Model. *Health Educ Q*. 1988;15(2):175–183.

10. Prochaska JO, DiClemente CC, Norcross JC. In search of how people change. Applications to the addictive behaviors. *Am Psychol*. 1992;47(9): 1102–1114.

11. Texas Department of State Health Services. Texas Yes You Can clinical toolkit for tobacco dependence.http://www.dshs.state.tx.us/tobacco/toolkit.shtm. Accessed February 25, 2010.

12. Bandura A. *Social Foundations of Thought and Action: A Social Cognitive Theory*. Englewood Cliffs, NJ: Prentice-Hall;1986.

13. Green LJ, Kreuter MW. Eds. *Health promotion planning: An Educational Ecological Approach*. New York, NY: McGraw Hill Companies, Inc; 2005.

14. U.S. Department of Health & Human Services. 2008 Physical activity guidelines for Americans: be active, healthy, and happy. www.health.gov/paguidelines. Accessed February 25, 2010.

15. Maibach E, Parrott RL. Eds. *Designing Health Messages: approaches from Communication Theory and Public Health Practice*. Thousand Oaks, CA: Sage Publications, Inc; 1995.

16. Bunge M, Mühlhauser I, Steckelberg A. What constitutes evidence-based patient information? Overview of discussed criteria. *Patient Educ Couns*. 2010;78(3):316–328. doi:10.1016/j.pec.2009. 10.029

17. Evans MW Jr. The ABC's of health promotion and disease prevention in chiropractic practice. *J Chiropr Med*. 2003;2(3):107–110.

18. Fiore MC, Jaén CR, Baker TB, et al. *Treating Tobacco Use and Dependence: Quick Reference Guide for Clinicians 2008 Update*. Rockville, MD: U.S. Department of Health and Human Services. The Public Health Service; 2009.

19. Ndetan HT, Bae S, Evans MW Jr, et al. Characterization of health status and modifiable risk behavior among United States adults using chiropractic care as compared to general medical care. *J Manipulative Physiol Ther*. 2009; 32(6):414–422.

20. Kreuter MW, Chheda SC, Bull FC. How does physician advice influence patient behavior? Evidence of a priming effect. *Arch Fam Med*. 2000;9(5):426–433.

21. Evans MW Jr, Hawk, C, Strasser SM. An educational campaign to increase chiropractic intern advising roles on patient smoking cessation. *Chiropr Osteopat*. 2006;14:24. doi:10.1186/1746-1340-14-24.

CHAPTER 3

Principles of Wellness Coaching

Cheryl Hawk

Health and wellness coaching is gaining both popularity and credibility as a method to assist people in successfully changing health behaviors. The International Coach Federation (ICF), the organization dealing with credentialing of coaches, has defined coaching as "partnering with clients in a thought-provoking and creative process that inspires them to maximize their personal and professional potential."[1] The perspective of coaching is client centered, focusing on the client actively setting goals and working to achieve them. Its perspective is *not* that of the practitioner, which would focus on providing the client with care or imparting information.

Coaching is also quite distinct from therapeutic counseling.[2] As summarized in Table 3.1, in general, conventional therapists usually focus on helping clients or patients identify areas in their life that are dysfunctional and examine their past to discover how the dysfunction developed. This comparison is used only to contrast general approaches, because many individual therapists also use many of the approaches described in this chapter. In fact, psychologists, psychotherapists, and counselors founded most of the techniques used in wellness coaching.[2] Coaches focus on the client's present strengths and skills, and based on these, help the client develop a plan to reach the expressed future goals. The focus on positive attributes and strengths and an orientation toward action and goal setting are the core of coaching, which distinguishes it from therapy and counseling. Integral to this approach is the concept that the coach does *not* operate as an "expert"; the coach facilitates the client's ability to find his or her own answers within.

The term "health coaching" is often applied to assisting clients with existing conditions to better manage them, whereas "wellness coaching" is applied to assisting healthy clients achieve optimal health and wellness. However, in actuality, there is much overlap between the two terms. The professions of health and wellness coaching are growing fast, due to the public's growing interest in self-care as well as employers' and insurance companies' awareness of the health care savings that can be achieved by reducing obesity, tobacco use, and other poor lifestyle choices.

It is becoming increasingly common for human resource departments or insurance companies to utilize coaches and/or health educators, usually for phone consultations, to assist their employees or insurance clients to modify their lifestyles. Busy health care providers may also wish to either employ a coach or refer their patients to one. However, many health care providers may also want to use coaching techniques to increase the effectiveness of their own counseling with patients. Although wellness coaching sessions are often structured to run 30 to 60 minutes, the techniques for assisting clients with behavior change can also

TABLE 3.1	Coaching Versus Counseling/Therapy
Coaching	**Counseling/Therapy**
Client finds his or her own answers	Counselor provides expert advice
Deals with client's present	Deals with client's past
Action-oriented	Feeling/emotion-oriented
Adult learning model: How to attain goals	Medical model: Diagnose and treat disease/dysfunction
Focus on present strengths and future goals	Focus on past events to resolve present pain and conflict

be used effectively in shorter time frames, as appropriate to most clinical settings. This chapter is not intended to substitute for in-depth wellness coach training, such as those programs credentialed by the ICF, the leading organization that provides standards and certification for the coaching profession (www.coachfederation.org).

This chapter introduces the principles of wellness coaching as they can be applied in a typical practice. Since it has been shown that counseling by family physicians is effective for helping patients change health behavior,[3] such counseling may also be expected to increase the effectiveness of the clinical encounter for other types of practitioners, in terms of optimal patient wellness.

THEORETICAL BASIS OF WELLNESS COACHING

Various models of organizational behavior and change have influenced the development of coaching. Coaching has been used extensively in business and other types of organizations to improve the efficiency and effectiveness of their employees.[2] However, its chief influences have been in the area of counseling psychology, particularly positive psychology.[4] This relative newcomer to psychological theories, initiated in 1998 by Martin Seligman, arose from the humanistic psychology movement.[5,6] Positive psychology, rather than focusing on pathology and negative emotions, focuses on positive emotions such as optimism, hope, courage, and spirituality, and on positive qualities—people's strengths, talents, and creativity.[6] Another important influence on wellness coaching is the Transtheoretical Model, which was described in Chapter 2.[7] Social Cognitive Theory, specifically the concept of self-efficacy,[8] also described in Chapter 2, contributes to wellness coaching theory as well.

A counseling approach that is often adapted to wellness coaching is motivational interviewing (MI). MI is considered a semidirective method that is particularly well suited to clients with addictive behaviors, especially those who have not yet considered making a health behavior change.[2,9,10] As this approach, which is more of a methodology than a model, was not discussed in Chapter 2, we will summarize it here. MI seeks to encourage clients to move toward changing their behavior through the following four principles:

1. *Express empathy*, which is based on the concept that acceptance helps encourage the client to change.

2. *Develop discrepancy*, which means that the counselor helps clients recognize the discrepancy between how they would like their lives to be and how they currently are; this cognitive dissonance fosters the client's own desire to change.

3. *Roll with resistance*, which means that the counselor accepts the client's current resistance to change as a natural stage, rather than opposing it, which would build greater resistance and not allow the client to develop motivation from within.

4. *Support self-efficacy*, which is essential for successful and lasting change.[9,10]

Applications of these theories and approaches will be discussed in the following sections of this chapter.

The Coach's Attitude

The first and most important thing a coach can do—especially one who is also a physician or health care provider—is to take off his expert hat. Coaching is not about imparting information; it is about empowering the client to make the change that he or she has selected. This is perhaps the most difficult part of coaching for health care professionals who have spent years becoming experts in their field! However, it is essential for successful coaching. Coaches need to do much more listening than talking, and more asking of questions than answering them. Your attitude as a coach must be that your client has all the information and ability already within that will be needed to make the desired life change. Your job is to help the client bring those necessary elements into awareness and action.

Coaching Techniques

Derived from the theories and approaches described above, a number of techniques are commonly used in wellness coaching. These are summarized in Table 3.2; they are open-ended questioning, appreciative inquiry, reflective listening, positive reframing, expressing empathy, working with decisional balance, and supporting self-efficacy.

OPEN-ENDED QUESTIONING

Open-ended questions are ones that do not have a "preset" answer, and so require more than one or two words to answer. Using open-ended questions is tremendously important in empowering the patient to find his or her own goals,

TABLE 3.2	Summary of Wellness Coaching Techniques
Technique	**How to Use It**
Open-ended questioning (also called open-ended inquiry)	Ask a question with no fixed response. Avoid "yes/no" questions!
Appreciative inquiry	Focus on the client's strengths rather than problems.
Reflective listening	Paraphrase what the client said. You may also amplify it to help the client gain insight.
Positive reframing	Reinterpret the client's statement in a positive way.
Expressing empathy	Demonstrate understanding and respect for the client's experience.
Working with decisional balance	Assist the client to list the pros and cons of behavior change.
Supporting self-efficacy	Help the client set small, attainable goals and develop a positive, "can-do" attitude.

motivators, and strategies for change.[11,12] These questions give control of the conversation to the client, rather than to the doctor. They are non-judgmental, since there is no "right" answer. In addition, they foster self-discovery and independence, promoting the patient's ownership of the process of change.

REFLECTIVE LISTENING

Reflective listening is one of the most basic and important tools in a coach's toolbox. You simply restate what the patient said, being careful to withhold judgment or interpretation. A prelude to a reflective listening statement is often, "So what I hear you saying is. . . ." This technique shows the patient that you are listening. Being listened to and heard is in and of itself a healing experience for most people. Also, this technique allows the patient to hear their own words, which often helps bring insight. Don't be concerned that you may be misinterpreting the patient's meaning, because reflecting back what you thought was said gives the patient an opportunity to clarify it, which is also helpful in developing insight.

POSITIVE REFRAMING

Positive reframing is an even more active technique than reflective listening. With this technique, the coach encourages the client who has expressed a negative attitude toward an experience to change his or her perspective to a positive one. Rather than viewing a lapse from his or her wellness plan as a failure, the client is urged to see it as "practice" from which he or she has gained valuable insights on how to succeed. "What did you learn from this experience?" is a good question to

help a client to positively reframe an experience he or she has been expressing negatively.

APPRECIATIVE INQUIRY

Appreciative inquiry is one of the coaching techniques that originated in the field of organizational behavior, although it is now commonly used in all types of counseling as well.[13] Completely counter to traditional schools of thought that focus on the etiology of emotional problems from past trauma, appreciative inquiry focuses on the client's strengths and on possibilities for success in the future, emphasizing positive emotions and a positive attitude.[2]

With this technique, the coach encourages the client to acknowledge and amplify his or her personal strengths rather than dwell on problems and weaknesses. Appreciative inquiry fosters a positive attitude toward the future and reframes the present in a positive manner. Imagining a positive future in which one's goals are realized is part of the process; this technique has much to do with the development of vision statements as a core component of the wellness plan.

EXPRESSING EMPATHY

Empathy is an essential part of any clinical encounter, but it is especially crucial to successful coaching. Empathy means that the coach both respects and understands the client's experience and frame of mind. This requires being non-judgmental, engaged, yet not being drawn into the client's drama—the coach must avoid sympathy, in which he or she identifies with the client's emotions and thus cannot effectively function as a coach. To convey a nonjudgmental attitude, both the coach and client make observations rather than evaluations. For example, it is an evaluation to say, "You should have exercised five days last week," or "I completely blew my exercise plan and only got to the gym once." It is an observation to say, "I exercised one time last week."

WORKING WITH DECISIONAL BALANCE

Enabling decisional balance is especially useful for clients who are still ambivalent about changing their health behavior. This technique entails simply listing the pros and cons of making the behavior change under consideration. Research indicates that people are moved from earlier stages of change, such as from precontemplation to contemplation, when their list of "pros" exceeds their list of "cons."[14] In addition, one can use a "readiness to change" ruler, anchored by "not ready to change" and "very ready to change" in conjunction with the list of pros and cons.[2,14] Rulers can be used for confidence and willingness to change, as well as readiness, to provide additional information. Figure 3.1 illustrates a readiness-to-change ruler.

SUPPORTING SELF-EFFICACY

The first step in developing the client's self-efficacy is for the coach to help her or him set attainable goals. This will enable the client to succeed, which will stimulate further successes. One way to assess whether the client's goals are reasonable is to use a simple "confidence scale." Ask the client, "On a scale of 0 to 10, how confident are you that you can reach this goal (in the specified time frame)?" Expert coaches say that if the client's score is 7 or higher, success is likely.[2] It is helpful to ask the client, "Why did you pick a '6' instead of a '5'?" Asking why he picked a "6" instead of

a "7" focuses on his shortcomings rather than his strengths. However, after finding out why he chose the higher number, it is often helpful to follow up by asking, "What do you think you might do, or what would have to happen, for this to be a '7' instead of a '6'?" This gets the client to consider how to take positive action forward, based on an awareness of his current strengths.

Self-efficacy is one of the most important factors in behavior change. Coaches need to support the client's self-efficacy in every way possible, and at every stage of coaching. The concept of self-efficacy was originally developed as part of Bandura's Social Cognitive Theory.[8] Bandura's theory posited that there are four approaches to reinforcing self-efficacy: Physiological or emotional states, verbal persuasion, vicarious experience, and mastery experience.

Physiological or emotional states refer to stimuli a person experiences. Experiencing distress— too much or not enough stimulation—decreases self-efficacy, while experiencing eustress ("good" stress) supports self-efficacy. Clinicians, particularly those who provide manual therapies, can greatly assist patients with their physiological stress response. Further, assisting them to recognize their stress level through coaching will amplify that influence. It is essential that clients or patients feel challenged and excited by their wellness journey, but it is also crucial that they do not become overwhelmed with the challenge to the point of distress. Breathing exercises, yoga, meditation, and other mind–body techniques can promote self-efficacy in physiological states. When a client's habitual reaction to challenge is "I'm scared," or "I'm anxious," the coach can help him or her to positively reframe this response as "I'm excited." This can free many people to begin to enjoy challenges rather than fear them.

☐ 0	☐ 1	☐ 2	☐ 3	☐ 4	☐ 5	☐ 6	☐ 7	☐ 8	☐ 9	☐ 10

0 = not ready to change   10 = already changing

Interpreting the Readiness-to-Change Ruler
The following provides a general "rule of thumb" for assessing a patient's stage of change:
0–2: precontemplation
3–5: contemplation
6–9: contemplation/preparation
  10: action

Figure 3.1. Readiness-to-change ruler.

Verbal persuasion means that the coach helps the client become convinced that he or she can make the health behavior change, not that he persuades him or her of what he or she should or should not do. "My certainty is greater than your doubt"[2(p. 58)] should be the coach's attitude toward the client— not certainty about what the client should do, but certainty that he or she can do it. Communicating a belief that he or she can do it is what is required.

Vicarious experience simply means that the client can develop self-efficacy through role models or support groups, where he or she can begin to believe, "if they can do it, I can do it!"

Mastery experience means that success breeds success. When the client masters a small step on his or her journey, it builds self-efficacy. The coach can facilitate this by helping him or her see relapses as "practice," instead of "failures," and we all know that "practice makes perfect."

DEVELOPING A WELLNESS PLAN

The wellness plan is based on the patient's or client's assessment and their expressed interests. Figure 3.2 gives an example of a wellness plan, with instructions. The plan itself is a single-page document of which the client and coach should both retain a copy. Key elements of the wellness plan are described below.

Assessment: The Groundwork for a Wellness Plan

Most practitioners are trained in assessing patients for disease, symptoms, and dysfunction, and for identifying past and current comorbidities. A wellness assessment requires that you also collect information on risk factors for poor health outcomes and on lifestyle and health behavior. This information can easily be collected at the same time the usual history, examination, and assessment are done. Since wellness is a multidimensional concept, assessment should be holistic. It should include, at a minimum, information to identify risk factors for the most prevalent diseases and conditions (i.e., heart disease, cancer, stroke, and injuries); depression; stress; assessment of general health status; and positive health. Specific tools for accomplishing this are described and presented in Chapter 7, Wellness Assessment and Clinical Preventive Services.

In addition to information on past and current health habits and risk factors, you should assess patients' readiness to change health behavior. The concept of "readiness to change" was discussed in Chapter 2. Determining a patient's stage of change is essential to provide the most appropriate and individualized guidance. Individualized information is more successful in promoting behavior change, and it also allows the practitioner to use his or her time most effectively.[7,15]

The following section summarizes how to identify patients in each stage of change and how to most effectively counsel them.

READINESS-TO-CHANGE RULERS

As introduced above, there are many variations on the concept of the "readiness-to-change" or "willingness-to-change" ruler. Usually, this ruler is anchored on the left by "not ready to change" and on the right by "already changing" or "very ready to change."[14] Since many practitioners already use 0-to-10 scales for assessing patients' pain or function, we will illustrate this concept with the same scale. See Figure 3.1 for a sample ruler. It can give you a rough estimate of the patient's current stage of change. Remember, people can be, and usually are, in different stages for different behaviors, and also shift from one stage to another over time, for the same behavior. The doctor's or coach's job is to help the person shift to the right, toward change.

PRECONTEMPLATION: "I WON'T"

Precontemplators are not considering making the behavior change in question; however, the "I won't" type is very different from the "I can't" type (see Table 3.3).[2] The "I won't" type of precontemplator is one who is simply unwilling to change. He or she has either not considered the health behavior to be a problem, or is in denial that it is a problem. Exhorting this patient to change his or her behavior will only elicit resistance, not compliance. For a very harmful behavior like smoking, you should make your position clear, without being too prescriptive: "As your doctor, I need to tell you that the most important thing you can do for your health is to stop smoking." Studies have shown that advice from a doctor does influence people to quit. However, when the patient is very definite about not wanting to make a change, the doctor should express empathy and understanding ("I know it's hard to change, and it's OK that you aren't ready right now.") and move on, broaching the topic again periodically.

PRECONTEMPLATION: "I CAN'T"

There are two types of "I can't" precontemplators.[2] The first is being simply unaware of the importance of the health behavior. They may not be

My Wellness Plan _____ Date: _____

Your vision: How do you see yourself 6 months from now?

_____

Motivators (list)

_____   _____

_____   _____

Confidence—On a scale of 0 (no confidence) to 10 (complete confidence), how confident are you that you can achieve your vision?

❏ 0   ❏ 1   ❏ 2   ❏ 3   ❏ 4   ❏ 5   ❏ 6   ❏ 7   ❏ 8   ❏ 9   ❏ 10

Challenges (list)

_____   _____

_____   _____

Strengths (list)

_____   _____

_____   _____

Support (list)

_____   _____

_____   _____

Strategies (describe at least one)

_____

_____

GOALS
3-month goal:

[   ]

1-week goal:

[   ]

Figure 3.2. Wellness plan.

educated about the importance of muscle strength in preventing falls, or the large amounts of sugar and salt in processed foods. These patients need information that will show them how important the health behavior in question is. Be sure and give them short, easy-to-understand information sheets or brochures, and let them know that you can answer their questions.

The other type of "I can't" precontemplator feels unable to change—that it is just too difficult to even think about it.[2] These patients first need your empathy about the difficulty of changing,

TABLE 3.3	Working with the Stages of Change		
Stage	**How to Identify**	**Strategies to Move Forward**	**Questions to Ask**
Precontemplation	No intent to change	—	—
"I won't"	Unwilling or in denial	Empathy; follow up periodically	"What might happen that would let you know that this is a problem?"
"I don't know"	Unaware; lacks knowledge	Short brochures	
"I can't"	Unable; lacks confidence	Build confidence (appreciative inquiry)	"What would have to happen that would make you have to change?"
Contemplation	Considering making change in next 6 mo	Identify strengths	"How will you know when it's time to (change the behavior)?"
"I might"	No actions yet	Identify motivators	
Preparation	Plans to make change within next month	Wellness plan with SMART goals	"What are some of the benefits to you of making this change?"
"I will"	Already has plans	—	
Action	Has made some changes	Support and praise	"What has worked the best about your plan so far?"
"I am"	—	Positive reframing if lapses occur	
Maintenance	Behavior change has been in effect for at least 6 mo	Follow up with positive reinforcement	"What was your biggest challenge in making this change, and what was the best way you found to overcome it?"
"I still am"	—	Positive reframing if lapses occur	Relapses: "What did you learn from this practice experience that will help you next time?"
—	—	Support groups/networking	—

and at the same time, you must help them build confidence and self-efficacy. Appreciative inquiry is a good technique for confidence building. For example, you could ask a patient who is depressed and has chronic pain, "Tell me about the best day you've had since I saw you last week." It is essential that precontemplators begin to realize that they *do* have some good days, some successes! Peer support groups are also helpful to these patients. In addition, positive reframing is an essential part of dialogues with these patients.

CONTEMPLATION: "I MIGHT"

Patients who say they might want to change their behavior within the next 6 months are contemplators. They have not yet made concrete plans, but are considering making the change. Your job is to help them move into the next stage. This can be done by helping them identify their personal strengths that will help them overcome the challenges that may be holding them back; brainstorming is a useful technique here. Brainstorming is a technique in which both the client and the coach contribute ideas "off the top of their heads," in an informal and free-flowing exchange, which can identify creative, valuable solutions. They may also need help in discovering strong motivators toward action. Additionally, they may need more in-depth information to help them develop a workable plan of action. This is where the practitioner blends coaching with expert knowledge, so that the patient can make informed choices in developing this plan.

PREPARATION: "I WILL"

The stage of preparation is the one doctors are most familiar with and, in fact, usually expect to see with patients. Once they have resolved to act within the next month, it is time to proceed with the wellness plan, as described below. At this point, it may be helpful to help this patient think about how to set small, achievable goals to experience success, which will increase confidence and self-efficacy.

ACTION: "I AM"

Clinicians often leave patients on their own if they are in the action stage, where they are actually setting about changing their behavior. This is a mistake; they need praise and support at this stage because behavior change is always difficult. Additionally, many, if not most, people have relapses along the way. It is important that the doctor help them positively reframe these as learning experiences ("practice makes perfect") rather than see them negatively ("trial and error").

MAINTENANCE: "I STILL AM"

Patients who have been maintaining their behavior change for at least 6 months are in maintenance. You can help them continue to maintain the behavior by continuing to provide praise and positive feedback. These patients can share their success stories, serving as role models for others, in support groups, which in turn helps other patients with their wellness efforts.

Vision Statement

A client's vision statement is a detailed visualization of what he or she wants. This is a relatively long-range goal, generally about 6 months from the present. The goals through which he or she will reach the vision are short-term. It is essential that he or she visualizes what he or she wants—a positive vision—rather than what he or she *doesn't* want. The subconscious tends to be quite literal, and lives in the present—therefore, the vision should be as specific and concrete as possible, and always framed in the present tense, *never* in the future. For example, a client who is overweight might have a vision statement saying: "I am healthy and full of energy, wearing my favorite size 8 jeans,"

Motivators

Most clients need help in discovering the factors that will provide incentives to reach their vision. You should emphasize that there are no "right"

or "wrong" motivators—what one person might consider frivolous might be a very strong motivator to another. For example, wanting to fit into her size 6 jeans again might not sound like a "serious" motivator to the doctor, but to the patient, this is a very real and important reason to change his or her diet and exercise habits. You must take off your "doctor" hat and be a coach, and help the client explore the factors that energize him or her to make needed behavior changes.

Confidence

Using a confidence scale of 0 to 10 is instructive to the coach and helpful to the client. If the client starts off with a confidence rating of 7 or higher, you can assume that success is likely.[2] It is worthwhile to inquire into the client's reasoning, especially with lower confidence ratings, to make sure that the vision is realistic enough to be attainable. However, always inquire using positively framed, nonjudgmental, and open-ended questions: "I see you marked your confidence as 3. What made you choose a 3 instead of a 2?" This gives the client an opportunity to express his or her perceived strengths instead of her perceived shortcomings.

Challenges

Clients must consider the difficulties they will encounter in their wellness journey, to be prepared to overcome them. Positively framing problems or difficulties as "challenges" will help them maintain a positive attitude. Challenges may be situations (going out to eat for someone whose goal is a healthier diet), people (a spouse who can "eat anything and not gain weight" for a homemaker whose goal is to be 20 lb slimmer, and who prepares family meals), or habits (a smoker whose goal is to be tobacco free, who always has a cigarette with his morning coffee).

Strengths

Most people have learned to focus on their problems and weaknesses, especially when they think about a health behavior they know they need to change. This can detract from their self-efficacy and confidence, and make it harder to succeed. You can help them enhance their strengths to enable them to meet their challenges and reach their goals. For example, if your client wants to be tobacco-free, you can ask her about what worked well when she had previously quit smoking (and remind her that practice makes perfect). Or you can remind her that she has been able to be promoted in her challenging job, or that she has succeeded in raising her children—there are always many areas of life in which clients have been successful, and they can use the traits that helped them succeed in other areas to succeed with their health goal.

Support

The client's support network is usually friends and family. It's important that the client identify specifically which family members and friends can be expected to provide various types of support. For example, a client who wants to exercise more might identify a friend who can be an "exercise buddy," find that her husband is willing to watch the kids while she exercises, and that her dog might turn out to be the best exercise buddy of all!

Strategies

You should make sure the client understands what a strategy is: a specific plan designed to meet a certain challenge. It's important to develop these strategies during the planning phase of a behavior change, so they are available when the challenge occurs and so the person is able to remain on course. The more specific and simple the strategy is, the better. It is helpful to take a few minutes with your client to brainstorm strategies. Strategies are most successful if the client comes up with them himself or herself. Strategies imposed by the coach as prescriptions may stimulate resistance, especially with people dealing with addictive behaviors. Developing his or her own strategies, rather than being given them by the coach, gives the client ownership and increases his or her investment in pursuing them. An example of developing a strategy: Your client is developing a tobacco cessation plan and lists as one of his challenges the desire for a cigarette at his coffee break. You might say, "Can you think of some alternatives to that cigarette that you feel might help you overcome the urge to smoke?" Both of you together can come up with some possibilities: taking five deep breaths; going for a walk instead of standing in the break area with the other smokers; and chewing gum instead. He feels that taking a walk would work best because it would remove him from the habitual setting where he and others smoke. However, he has the other alternatives in mind as well, as fallback strategies.

Goals

Goals are what we use to reach our vision. It generally works well to have the client set initial 3-month and 1-week goals. Goals should be **SMART**: **S**pecific, **M**easurable, **A**ction-oriented, **R**ealistic, and **T**ime-framed. Most people will

pick up the SMART concept most easily if you give them examples.

After helping the client to develop the wellness plan, be sure to follow up at 1-week intervals and use the techniques described in this chapter to help him or her stay motivated and reach the 3-month goal. If his or her vision is a long-range one (which will often be the case for long-standing health challenges), the goals can then be reset for the next 3 months, to keep moving toward the vision.

Literature Cited

1. International Coach Federation. What is coaching? http://www.coachfederation.org/about-icf/overview/.
2. Moore M, Tschannen-Moran B. *Coaching Psychology Manual*. Philadelphia, PA: Wolters Kluwer; 2010.
3. Searight H. Realistic approaches to counseling in the office setting. *Am Fam Physician*. 2009;79(4):277–284.
4. Linley P, Harrington S. Positive psychology and coaching psychology: perspectives on integration. *The Coaching Psychologist*. 2005;1(1):1–3.
5. Stober DR, Grant AM. *Evidence-based Coaching Handbook*. Hoboken, NJ: John Wiley & Sons; 2006.
6. Seligman ME, Csikszentimihalyi M. Positive psychology. An introduction. *Am Psychologist*. 2000;55(1):5–14.
7. Prochaska JO, Velicer WF. The transtheoretical model of health behavior change. *Am J Health Promotion*. 1997;12(1):38–48.
8. Bandura A. *Social Foundations of Thought and Action: a Social Cognitive Theory*. Englewood Cliffs, NJ: Prentice-Hall; 1986.
9. Miller WR, Rollnick S. *Motivational Interviewing: Preparing People for Change*. 2nd ed. New York, NY: Guilford Press; 2002.
10. Rollnick S, Miller WR, Butler C. *Motivational Interviewing in Health Care: Helping Patients Change Behavior*. New York, NY: Guilford Press; 2008.
11. Hecht J, Borrelli B, Breger RK, Defrancesco C, Ernst D, Resnicow K. Motivational interviewing in community-based research: experiences from the field. Ann Behav Med. 2005 Apr;29 Suppl:29-34.
12. Resnicow K, Dilorio C, Soet JE, et al. Motivational interviewing in health promotion: it sounds like something is changing. *Health Psychol*. 2002;21(5):444–451.

13. Cooperrider D, Whitney, D. *Appreciative Inquiry: a Positive Revolution in Change*. San Francisco, CA: Berrett-Koehler; 2005.

14. Zimmerman GL, Olsen C, Bosworth MF. A 'stages of change' approach to helping patients change behavior. *Am Fam Physician*. 2000;61(5):1409–1416.

15. Anspaugh D, Hamrick MH, Rosato FD. *Wellness: Concepts and Applications*. 7th ed. Boston, MA: McGraw-Hill; 2009.

CHAPTER 4

Health Communications in the Clinical Setting

Marion W. Evans, Jr.

First, let us concede that health communications is a very broad, well-researched discipline that is the primary subject of many a textbook dedicated solely to the topic. In the case of this chapter, the information provided is tailored to clinicians in the office environment. The typical patient comes to the office with a chief complaint. That is, they have some ailment or condition that they have determined needs your expert attention. Since this book is specifically focused on dealing with advising patients on wellness and promotion of health, that means the authors feel it takes a unique skill set to be effective in communicating on such topics through the acute pain or routine care visit. Of course there are opportunities to advise patients when they are not in the office for an acute care visit, and that is also within the scope of this chapter but for the most part, clinicians need to be cognizant of the fact that the patient may not be focused on hearing a prevention message if they are in pain or not feeling well. Since knowledge is necessary, even though some have said not "sufficient" for behavior change, communicating the message is a critical piece of the doctor–patient relationship that needs to start off on the right footing for the greatest chance of success. Hence, health communications has been defined as "the way [one] seeks, processes, and shares health information."[1]

Think about how you currently greet and listen to your patient on a typical first visit. Do you listen attentively and wait for him or her to complete the history? Do you allow this to develop in a distraction-free environment? How about encouraging a patient to write down any questions that arise after the visit and bring them back next time for discussion? It may be of interest to the reader to know that researchers in a study of doctor–patient communications found that on average, a primary care physician interrupted the patient within the first 22 seconds of intake.[2] Had the physician not interrupted the patient, within 2 minutes on average, the patient would have finished what he or she had to say. Rhoades and colleagues[3] also found more than doctor-evoked interruptions in the clinical setting. Computer use, pagers, knocks at the door all played a role in decreasing the effectiveness of communications. Residents were worse than physicians, with new residents interrupting patients most frequently; at times, within 12 seconds of entering the room!

A study on low back pain found that older patients received less information about their condition, as did those with chronic conditions.[4] In addition, one in three Americans may be functionally illiterate. To complicate this picture, most people simply do not comprehend medical terminology that has taken years for the typical clinician to accumulate. For these reasons, clinical health care providers need to take time to develop a better understanding of how to communicate health messages to patients. This can enhance patient satisfaction, lead to better follow-through on provider recommendations, and leave less room for error or misunderstanding in the clinical encounter. This should also be considered part of the informed consent process.

THE INITIAL PATIENT ENCOUNTER

In any clinical setting, one is likely to hear a doctor meeting a patient or a family member for the first time state something like, "Hello, I'm Dr X." But what about the patient's perspective on that matter? A recent study of initial introductions by doctors and patients found some surprising facts about this tone-setting introduction. First, a slight majority of patients (56%) preferred that the doctor introduce himself or herself by the first and last names, rather than by title.[5] They also preferred a handshake. Why not state to the patient, "I'm John Smith, your doctor . . .?" Furthermore, patients felt a more personal relationship with their provider when the provider called them by their first name rather than Mr. or Mrs. If this is not the case, patients will likely inform the provider by telling him or her their name, by use of Mr. or Mrs. It is possible, however, that introductions of a more personal nature remove a barrier to doctor–patient communications right from the beginning. In another study of patients' preferences for a doctor's appearance, researchers found that patients did not mind being addressed by their first names, but generally preferred the doctor introduce themselves as "Doctor" so there is no general rule of thumb on the topic. It is something to think about as you try to communicate better with your patients from day one of their clinical experience. A final word about introductions: There may be cultural or other differences based upon geographic location, and it is the provider's responsibility to be sensitive to these.

As the provider meets with the patient for the first time and is listening carefully to what he or she has to say, it is important to think about what the patient needs to know to successfully carry out doctor's orders. What are the dos and don'ts for the typical conditions seen in your office? Do you communicate those with the patient verbally, in writing, or both? It is probably a good idea to have prepared take-home information on how patients can follow through with your recommendations. There are some general rules on reading levels for information that must be read as well. That will follow later in this chapter.

It is important to know about the boundaries of personal space and other cultural norms. For example, it is a general rule of thumb that if you are standing any closer to a patient than 18 inches, you have typically invaded his or her personal space. It is best to keep a greater distance than this between you and the patient unless the clinical visit requires less. Remember, in this case we are talking about initial introductions and communications and not a prostate exam. In some cultures, such as in most of Europe or the United States, eye-to-eye contact is considered good communication. In other cultures this is not true. If you practice in areas where there is a great deal of diversity, it is always good to know the cultural differences and be aware of what your patients prefer.

In general, the typical patient wants to know the following as a minimum:

- That the doctor knows about their case and conditions
- What they should do to help assist in getting well
- What they shouldn't do that may interfere with getting well

- What your treatment will do, and what it will not do
- Side effects of treatment and when they should be alarmed or call you back
- That the doctor feels empathy for them
- General dos and don'ts for home, work, and play
- Options to the treatment you are recommending including watchful waiting

It is important to remember that in today's connected world, if clinicians do not cover all the information the patient may need, the patient will just go to the Internet. With the variation in reliability of information on the web, that may not be a good thing when it comes to health care advice.

Types of Doctor–Patient Communication

Four models of doctor–patient relationships have been detailed in the health care literature.[6] These include the following types of relationships: Paternalistic, scientific, collegial, and contractual. Each one has different characteristics and may be favored by some patients but if the doctor–patient relationship is to be a partnership, some will have more desirability than others. In all, patient autonomy should be maintained at all costs.

Paternalistic: This is an older, less partnership-oriented model in which essentially the doctor knows best, advises the patient what to do, and he or she does it without asking questions (or going on the Internet!)

Scientific: The doctor presents information to the patient with a full range of treatment options, and the patient makes choices based on direction given by the doctor. After all, aren't doctors scientists?

Collegial: The doctor uses the same premise as in the scientific model but acts more as a counselor to the patient. The doctor gives less direction and the patient has more autonomy.

Contractual: The doctor helps the patient in the decision-making process and attempts not only to counsel, but also to empower the patient to act in his or her own best interests. This is the "physician as teacher" model.

One can see that this ranges from a paternalistic doctor stating, "Lose 30 pounds before I see you next time," providing no resources, to a collegial or contractual model where the doctor is empathetic, listens to the patient's concerns, discusses the best way to approach a needed change or problem, provides links to resources and established goals, and appropriate follow-up. As stated, some patients may prefer one model or another, but a model in which the patient's best interests are front and center should be the model of choice. Autonomy, patient knowledge of what to do, and anything one can do to empower that patient to make successful changes in health status should be the goal of all clinicians.

THE REPORT OF FINDINGS

Flocke and Stange[7] evaluated over 2,600 adult outpatient visits in 138 family physician offices in 84 practices. They measured the provisions of health behavioral advice through direct observation. Recall rates varied but one thing was for certain: Patients presenting for acute care recalled less. But if a health behavior was needed to respond to a specific health condition for which the patient was being seen, there was an associated two fold increase in patient recall. Emphasizing the relevance to the patient and his or her current condition of the needed behavior change in your report of findings is very important. For example, those with an acute health problem that could be related to diet were more likely to recall if dietary advice was given as a means of helping that condition. For the most part, the more time spent discussing the behavior, the more likely the patient was to recall it. That does not mean every patient needs a mini-seminar, but the time a doctor spends with a patient over a few visits can add up if health messages are concentrated on what should be done to reach a greater level of health. It is also a good practice to ask patients to write down the questions that come up after the visit; but only if you really will discuss those with them at their next visit.

What Your Patient Needs to Hear

In a report of findings, patients are often distracted. They may be uncomfortable, in pain, afraid, confused by medical terminology as has been stated, and overwhelmed with new information. The best outcome of the report of findings is that your patient will understand what you want him or her to do, be successful in follow-through (that includes keeping your appointment), and will get better.

In your report of findings, a patient needs to hear the following:

- What is wrong?
- How can you help?
- How long until I feel better?

- What can I do to help get me better faster?
- What might I be doing to complicate my own clinical picture?
- How can I successfully follow through?

It is always best to start with simple concepts and explain those, moving gradually to the more complex. Avoid polysyllabic words if possible. The more polysyllables you use, the higher the grade reading level and the less an average patient will understand. Be empathetic, let them know you see the condition a lot and can help but only if this is true. Pay attention to cultural norms and differences. Don't blame patients for their condition. Studies on victim-blaming are known to discourage patients and will not improve progress.

It is also a good idea to reiterate what you covered at the end of your report and plan to do this again when they are out of pain or feeling better. And remember to tie any behavior change to the condition they have at the moment. For instance, if they smoke and have lower back pain, make them aware that smoking increases the risk of their spinal problem becoming chronic, not to mention the other negatives associated with tobacco use. A typical patient may recall less than 50% of what was said immediately after leaving the doctor's office.[8] Making communications a key feature of your practice style is critical to helping your patient achieve maximum results.

LITERACY LEVELS AND HEALTH CARE

As our population in the United States ages, hearing and memory issues will also become more problematic for many patients. Poor health literacy is likely to complicate this picture. You will learn more about this in subsequent chapters, but what we know about general literacy in America is not good. More than one-third of patients aged 65 and older have poor health literacy, and as many as 80% of hospitalized patients experience this.[9] This can have a negative effect on your ability to help your patient get well and this cannot be overstated. In a patient-centered environment, every effort should be made to help patients understand what is expected of them and how they can assist in their own health care. Anytime it is possible and allowable, with a patient in a new environment or with a new problem we encourage another family member to be present when findings or instructions are explained. This is simply good health care.

Many Americans cannot read, write, speak English and function in society at a successful level. The issue of health literacy is even worse.

Many cannot understand or function in a medical or health care environment well enough to take home messages about what has been done, needs to be done to them, or what they need to do to follow doctors' orders. *Healthy People 2010* defined health literacy as "The degree to which individuals have the capacity to obtain, process and understand basic health information and services needed to make appropriate health decisions."[10] Americans, on average, read at about the fifth- or sixth-grade level. When it comes to health issues, this level may be even lower.[11] Therefore, it is probably best to be at or below the fifth-grade reading level with anything your patient takes out of the office to read later. Forms in your office should probably take this into account as well. Since the invention of the personal computer there have been tools to assess documents, and in the case of Microsoft Word there is a readability tool built right in. This can be accessed as follows:

- Select "Review" on the Windows tool bar
- Select "Spelling and Grammar" from the tools tab at left
- Select "Options" in the lower left corner
- Check the box labeled "Show readability statistics" (under the heading "When correcting spelling and grammar in Word" about halfway down the box)

Once this is done, each time you spell- and grammar-check your document, you will receive a reading grade level of what you have written. You may also want to copy and paste a paragraph or two from your current office brochures or materials into Word and try this as well. The SMOG readability assessment protocol for a written sample appears as Table 4.1. This tool can be applied to materials that were written elsewhere. Remember, reading level assessments are not the end-all of your evaluation of readability. The information needs to make sense for the audience at which it is being aimed. For this reason it is a good idea to have staff, family, or even current patients read the material and get feedback from them prior to actual use in the office.

COMMUNICATING WITH OTHER PROVIDERS

Communication is not limited to the doctor–patient interface. We interact with other entities, health insurance companies, diagnostic centers, and providers as well. Regardless of the provider you may be working with for the overall benefit

TABLE 4.1	SMOG Readability Assessment

To calculate the reading grade level of a document, start with the complete document in front of you. Follow these steps:

Count 10 consecutive sentences near the beginning, the middle, and the end of your document

From these 30 sentences, circle the polysyllabic words (containing three or more syllables), including words with polysyllables that appear more than once in a sentence

Total the number of polysyllabic words

Estimate the square root of the total number of words that are polysyllabic by finding the nearest perfect square root to that number

Add a constant of 3 to the square root. The resulting number is the SMOG grade or reading level for the document

There are also calculators available online that allow the user to put in the number of polysyllabic words and receive an automatic calculation

Source: From McLaughlin G. SMOG grading: a new readability formula. *J Reading.* 1969;12(8):639–646, with permission.

of the patient, a good line of communication is always an important item for the patient's well-being. Keep in mind that the patient's consent to contact other providers is not only paramount to good communications, but is also required under new laws governing health care privacy. It will be critical to know what they prefer when it comes to communicating with other providers. For example, if the patient has a primary care doctor, it is always prudent to inform him or her of what is going on with your care if you are functioning as a specialist. If you are a primary care contact for the patient, you may be in touch with various specialty offices and therefore, will need to provide pertinent information relative to the patient's health status.

Writing a letter to the patient's other provider should be concise unless you are conveying complex medical information related to the case. A letter stating that the patient has been seen, what they have been seen for, and the treatment goals and prognosis is probably a minimal courtesy that should be extended, as long as the patient consents to this in advance. Consent should be recorded in writing within the patient chart. At times, when a referral for specialty diagnostic workup is made, the information may need to be of a more complex nature, and that may take the form of a narrative report, which is beyond the scope of this chapter. A follow-up letter to the referring or primary care doctor stating the patient has made progress should also be considered part of the routine process of communication.

In any letter to another provider, it is best to include the following:

- Language common to all providers
- The diagnostic code for which you are treating the patient
- All specific treatments you are providing
- An initial goal or prognosis
- Your willingness and availability to discuss the case
- A spell and grammar check!!

MESSAGE FRAMING

Gain-Framing For Positive Effects

Message framing has been mentioned in Chapter 2 on health behavioral theory but is worth mentioning again. When the doctor is providing messaging to a patient about what is wrong, what the patient must do, and what the hoped-for outcome is for treatment, it is generally best to gain-frame the message. That is, tell the patient what the benefits of care and home instructions are and what they gain from following through, rather than the negatives of not doing so.

Fear-Appeals

In some cases fear-appeals have been used in which the doctor attempts to scare the patient into taking the needed actions to better their health. This is a loss-frame perspective, and such appeals have been used in a variety of public health messaging campaigns, generally emphasizing the harmful physical effects or social consequences of failing to comply with health recommendations.[13–15] They are used in approximately 25% of public service announcements aimed at getting people to change behaviors. Perhaps the most popular ad used a frying pan, an egg, and the announcer suggesting that the frying egg was "your brain on drugs." Many will recall this message used sometime after the War on Drugs era in public service messages related to drug abuse prevention. Although we do not suggest these as the initial modes of communicating a health message to patients, with some patients they may be motivators when other

attempts have failed. In all, it is better to discuss the positive gains that will be made by adhering to a partnership with your office than trying to scare patients into the direction you wish them to go.

At times, patients may not perceive themselves to be at risk. For example, as our population has become heavier, many people who are overweight perceive themselves to be normal because so many people are overweight. In this case, it is important to make sure the patient is truly aware of what his or her actual risk is, especially if the perception is different from reality. This does not mean that you shouldn't tell patients the truth about their condition or its prognosis. Simply put, when you can accentuate the positive that a health behavior change will make, patients can be more receptive. However, if you must put the fear of reality into them, one phenomenon that can occur when such fear-appeals are used inappropriately is that people will simply deny that the message applies to them. This is referred to as *defensive avoidance*. Therefore, messages that are successfully planted using this method must not put too much fear into the patient and must have a realistic risk associated with them. The patient must have the self-efficacy to make needed changes or fear-appeals may only be worrisome and make him or her feel more vulnerable to the risk at hand. The two basic necessities of a successful fear-based message are (1) The message must include a threat of severe physical harm or social harm if the patient does not comply with recommendations (now, this should be true and not exaggerated) and (2) this risk must be personalized to the particular patient and must not be a general threat. Again, patients must feel they can successfully respond to the threat and that they have the skills to follow through on the specific recommendations made to reduce the risk. It is still recommended that one gain-frame messages where it is possible, but never reduce a patient's real health threat to less than what it actually is, and be truthful about where he or she stands even if the prognosis is poor.

Patient-Centeredness

Patient-centered care is about truthful relationships with every patient. It is also about expressing a patient's actual risks when he or she is in need of lifestyle-related behavior change, to empower the patient to make health improvements. Communication of risks begins with making a person aware of his or her actual, personal risk factors. This should be followed by helping patients acknowledge that the risks are factual and that they should perceive them as such, encouraging them to accept the need to make changes and then adhere to those behaviors or lifestyle-related changes once they have been made. It is also about weighing the risk versus benefits related to any care that is being rendered and making sure patients fully understand this ratio.

DIFFUSION AND ADOPTION OF NEW INFORMATION

Are you among the first in your group to purchase the latest smart phone or computer technology? How about the latest medical software? For some of us adoption of new technology is threatening and to others, we simply have to have it now! Rogers[15] developed a model related to how information diffuses into society and this can be translated into communication with patients. First, Rogers said "adoption" of new ideas or devices occurs in a bell-shaped curve distribution of five categories of people. These are innovators, early adopters, early majority adopters, late majority adopters, and laggards. If you are a laggard, you know who you are.

Innovators are those who stand in line to get the newest technology as it is unveiled at the Apple Store, and early adopters, early majority, late majority follow in a bell curve distribution (Fig. 4.1). In that distribution, innovators lie out to the left on the flat part of the curve representing fewer people as do laggards who are out in the flat part of the right side of the distribution. What

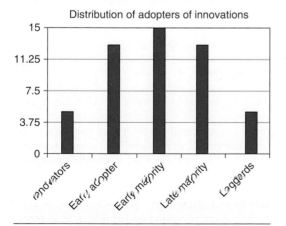

Figure 4.1. Distribution of adopters of new innovations based on Rogers.

Source: From Rogers EM. *Diffusion of Innovations*. 4th ed. New York, NY: Free Press; 2003, with permission.

is known about how new technology "diffuses" into a society can indeed be helpful in communications. First, think about what makes innovators or early adopters different. Do they do their homework and know something before everyone else does? Probably; and they are also likely to be curious people who are always wanting to know more. However, not everyone is like that. Rogers[16] said that for a person to want to try something new (let's say a new form of treatment in this case, or to change to a new behavior) they needed to know a few things. The "relative advantage" is the first thing. That is, what is the advantage of doing one thing versus another over, say, simply doing nothing? Translated, what is the advantage of changing to a healthier behavior? Next, is it "compatible" with what they perceive their needs to be or, in some cases, with who they are? Does it fit them? In the case of the construct "complexity," Rogers thought that if it was difficult to follow through on something, people would be less likely to adopt it. How intuitive is it to perform a new behavior or how difficult is it to eat differently? These will weigh on the decision-making process for most people. The next consideration is "trialability." Simply put, can they try it out? Experiment with it? Can you propose a "trial treatment period" in which the patient can judge if a new treatment is working prior to continuing? And last, the construct of "observability." Can they observe tangible results? If so, how soon? This too will have an effect. The sooner people can see that what they are doing for themselves is working, the more likely they will be to "adopt" a new behavior. Physical activity is a good example. For most people, starting an exercise program today will not provide immediate results that are tangible for several weeks. It is important then to stress that lifestyle changes in physical activity levels will take some time before a patient sees a positive difference. Give them a time-frame if you can. This may help keep patients encouraged until the results are more visible. It is also important to set small, incremental goals within the patient's ability to reach as this helps build needed self-efficacy.

WEBSITES AND OTHER SOCIAL MEDIA

Today, perhaps more so than ever before, information is at the fingertips. Computers, smart phones, and television interfacing with computers are making information easy to get and easy to place in the hands of people who are looking for it. Health information is no different. However, as we have stated earlier, health literacy is a major issue. People simply don't understand health terminology. That doesn't mean they won't try to understand or self-diagnose on the Internet. This will likely become more common as the cost of smart phones declines and as more services and applications become available through television programming and the Internet. Today, many clinical practices also use the Internet to reach their market, which in the case of health care is patients—people. Unfortunately, when information has been evaluated on the Internet by health scientists, what those sites communicate is, more often than not, less desirable than it could be. It may range from the legitimate to the ridiculous.

Studies performed on what can be found on the Internet related to management of childhood fever, depression, scoliosis, back pain, and even "wellness and chiropractic" have found information to be of poor quality and in some cases, in conflict with current, acceptable public health, wellness, or medical information.[17–21] For this reason, we make a note of it here and render some advice on how to provide information on the web that people can use, but also to caution doctors who may be thinking of buying a canned website from vendors who may not know what they are talking about.

Health on the Net Foundation (www.hon.ch/) has established guidelines on what constitutes good health information on the web. The site lists eight things a website should have to be deemed appropriate and fair to patients.

1. Information should be authoritative, providing the qualifications of those giving the advice (authors).
2. The site should state clearly the purpose of the website.
3. The site owner should respect the confidentiality of the users, not divulging sensitive health information.
4. The information should be documented and supported, citing dates and sources of the information or advice given.
5. Claims should be justified.
6. Website contact details should be apparent.
7. Funding of the site should be disclosed.
8. An advertising policy should be stated that allows the user to distinguish between health information and editorial content or advertisements and marketing ploys.

Sites that are essentially marketing tools for doctors to get patients to "trade" personal information for more health information are unethical and should be avoided as they may also violate state board laws governing various health care practices. Information on the website should be directed at helping people get the care they need, should be truthful, and should not contradict accepted health information when such information exists. To do this is to undermine good doctor–patient communications before the patient even sets foot in the office. Ensure that information placed on Facebook, Twitter, websites, or other forms of social media has the patient's best interests in mind and not simply the marketing of services. Sources of good health information can be derived from websites such as the ones listed in Table 4.2. Remember, whether you say it or not, what you provide on the Internet is out there for the world to see and reflects on the type of provider you are. This is sending a message, a communication to patients or future patients whether you realize this or not, and it may be out there for years with what we currently know about the Internet. Be careful and truthful and you can't go wrong.

NONVERBAL COMMUNICATION

As we have stated, nonverbal communication involves anything that is not communicated through voice. How does your carpet look? Worn? Soiled? That says something about your practice. Did you wash or sanitize your hands before you touched your patient? Is the paper on your examination table wrinkled and dirty? If so, you may be sending a message to your patient you would rather they not have received.

We have discussed that introductions and early impressions are very important. We have discussed a bit about how people perceive messages, how they understand information, and the importance of literacy levels. Other forms of nonverbal communication include what patients see, how they perceive you upon first impression, your tone, office vibe, materials you have in the reception area, and anything else you do not verbally communicate to them. You should take into account that anything that is nonverbal is communicating a message to your patient. Are you overweight? Does your lab coat look clean? Do you or a staff member smoke and reek of cigarettes? What is playing on the TV in your reception room? Do you have a nice, well-lit waiting area with up-to-date magazines and helpful information about health and wellness? All of this either supports a message of health and wellness

TABLE 4.2	Helpful Websites and Links to Find Usable Informative Material in Wellness and Prevention for Your Website or Social Media
America's Health Rankings	www.americashealthrankings.org
American Heart Association	www.americanheart.org
American Public Health Association	www.apha.org
Body Mass Index Calculator and Tables	www.nhlbisupport.com/bmi
Bone and Joint Decade (Bone and Joint Health)	www.usbjd.org
The Community Guide to Preventive Services	www.thecommunityguide.org
County Health Rankings	www.countyhealthrankings.org
Familydoctor.org	http://familydoctor.org
Find a Farmer's Market	http://apps.ams.usda.gov/FarmersMarkets
Fruit and Veggies More Matters	www.fruitsandveggiematter.gov
HRSA Health Literacy site	www.hrsa.gov/healthliteracy
Institute of Medicine	www.iom.edu
Let's Move (1st Lady Michelle Obama's site)	www.letsmove.gov
My (Health) Pyramid	www.mypyramid.gov
National Cancer Institute	www.cancer.gov
National Institutes of Health	www.nih.gov
National Library of Medicine	www.nlm.nih.gov
2008 Physical Activity Guidelines for Americans	www.health.gov/paguidelines
Put Prevention Into Practice	http://www.ncbi.nlm.nih.gov/books/NBK16634
U.S. Centers for Disease Control and Prevention	www.cdc.gov
U.S. Centres for Disease Control and Prevention website widgets	www.cdc.gov/widgets/#available
Spark People (Diet and Menu Plans)	www.sparkpeople.com
Straighten Up America (Posture–Spine Health)	www.straightenupamerica.org
Trust for America's Health	www.healthyamericans.org
Wellness Council of America	www.welcoa.org
World Health Organization	www.who.int

or it doesn't. A list of favorable verbal and non-verbal communicative measures can been seen in Table 4.3. Try to apply them in everyday practice.

Dress Code

Nowadays doctors may wear scrubs, a dress shirt and tie or jeans. This probably has as much to do with geographic or local cultural variation, and we feel that as long as you look like the other professionals in your area, your appearance is probably acceptable to patients. However, with that said, here is a little research on the topic.

The history of the white coat goes back to the late 19th century and was meant to relay a "cloak of scientific validity" about the doctor as well as to represent purity and cleanliness.[23] However, the same historical paper on this topic admits that white coats can harbor germs and cross-contaminate, serve to intimidate patients, and even turn patients off if it is visibly soiled. In that commentary, authors reported that 65% of patients in the study thought a doctor should have a white coat on, and 37% thought a male should wear a necktie. Thirty-four percent thought females should wear a skirt; probably 34% of the 37% who thought males should wear a tie!

In 2005, a study of internal medicine clinics found that more than 75% of people favored

TABLE 4.3	Favorable Doctor–Patient Communications Attributes

Expression of empathy on the part of the doctor

Reassurance or support

Encouragement to ask questions

Allow the patient's point of view to be heard, expressed

Explanations

Laughing and joking (where appropriate)

Addressing problems the patient has with activities of daily living

Asking about stress-related or psychosocial issues

Increased time spent on health education with the patient

Sharing (explaining) medical data

Discussion of treatment effects

Friendliness

Courtesy

Receptive to questions and patient statements

Clarifying statements

Listening

Summarization on the patient's level

Increased encounter length

Orienting the patient to the physical examination

Source: From Beck RS, Daughtridge R, Sloane PD. Physician–patient communication in the primary care office: systematic review. *J Am Board Fam Pract.* 2002;15(1):25–38, with permission.

professional attire for doctors, followed by 10% or so thinking surgical scrubs more appropriate for today.[24] The remainder preferred professional business dress or thought it was acceptable to go casual. Respondents stated they were significantly more likely to share personal, health-related information with someone who looked professionally dressed.

An additional study from New Zealand found similar results related to professional attire, with more preferring it than not.[25] In this study, less formal dress was acceptable as long as the doctor was smiling. This was followed by a preference for a white coat, followed by traditional business attire, casual attire, and then jeans. The older the patient, the more likely they were to prefer a more formal doctorly look. While we emphasize that in today's culture, as long as you look like the other professionals in your area you are probably doing

fine; we also encourage you (males) not to wear worn jeans with a tobacco can ring in the back pocket. We have seen that in Texas and it does NOT relay a message that you care about anyone's health. Good grooming characteristics are also typically preferred, so you should look neat, composed, and clean. No one wants a slob for a doctor; no matter how good you are. Do your best to send positive, nonverbal as well as verbal communications that are going to be conducive to a healing environment.

Final Tips on Better Doctor–Patient Communications

du Pré[26] outlines some very practical tips for better communications with patients and care givers:

- Use open-ended questions and listen attentively until the patient is finished.
- Don't rush patients (or even appear to be rushed).
- Don't sit with your arms crossed.
- Avoid abrupt shifts in topic without a transition, such as cutting the patient off with an additional closed-ended question.
- Determine the main reason for the visit PRIOR to the examination.
- Listen for distress markers in the patient's voice, such as stuttering or other signs of stress, which may occur just before divulging more important information.
- Ask for feedback from your patient to make sure you are on the right track with what he or she is telling you.
- Reassure your patient.
- Treat them as equals in the relationship and earn their trust.
- Coach patients by helping them understand what you do, but in terms they can understand.
- Consider using humor when appropriate.

Verbal Tracking

Verbal tracking such as repeating in your own words what a patient has just said may also reassure him or her that you are listening. Asking for direct feedback related to the problem can do this as well, such as "If I understand you correctly, your pain is keeping you up at night and doesn't respond well to over-the-counter medicines . . ." or "From what you have told me, you experience bloating and gas after you eat mainly fried foods." Essentially, tracking is repeating what has been said in a way that lets the patient know you are listening and have understood what they have told you.

SUMMARY

Successful communication is critical in the doctor–patient encounter. It takes on many different aspects from direct verbalization to nonverbal communications, such as how one dresses, speaks, or presents oneself in an initial introduction. The importance of getting this communication right from the beginning is crucial to helping patients modify lifestyle through behavior change and keep them following through on doctors' orders that will move them toward better health outcomes.

Literature Cited

1. Kreps GL, Thornton BC. Health Communications: theory and Practice. 2nd ed. Prospect Heights, IL. Waveland Press; 1992:2.
2. Langewitz W, Denz M, Keller A, et al. Spontaneous talking time at start of consultation in outpatient clinic: cohort study. *BMJ*. 2002; 325(7366):682–683.
3. Rhoades DR, McFarland KF, Finch WH, et al. Speaking and interruptions during primary care office visits. *Fam Med*. 2001;33(7): 528–532.
4. Gulbrandsen P, Madsen HB, Benth JS, et al. Health care providers communicate less well with patients with chronic low back pain–a study of encounters at a back pain clinic in Denmark. *Pain*. 2010;150(3):458–461.
5. Makoul G, Zick A, Green M. An evidence-based perspective on greetings in medical encounters. *Arch Intern Med*. 2007;167(11):1172–1176.
6. Emanuel EJ, Emanuel LL. Four models of the physician-patient relationship. *JAMA*. 1992;267:2221–2226.
7. Flocke SA, Stange KC. Direct observation and patient recall of health behavior advice. *Prev Med*. 2004;38(3):343–349.
8. Ong LM, de Haes JC, Hoos AM, et al. Doctor–patient communication: a review of the literature. *Soc Sci Med*. 1995;40(7):903–918.
9. Williams MV, Davis T, Parker RM, et al. The role of health literacy in patient–physician communication. *Fam Med*. 2002;34(5):383–389.
10. United States Department of Health and Human Services. Healthy people 2010. http://www.healthypeople.gov/Document/pdf/uih/2010uih.pdf. Accessed January 25, 2010.
11. United States Department of Health and Human Services. The Public Health Service. Making Health Communications Work. , Bethesda, MD: National Cancer Institute, National Institute of Health; 2002. Publication No. 02-5145.
12. McLaughlin G. SMOG grading: a new readability formula. J Reading 1969;12(8):639–646.
13. Maibach E, Parrott RL. Designing Health Messages: approaches from Communication Theory and Public Health Practice. Thousand Oaks, CA: Sage; 1995: 65–79.
14. Millar MG, Millar KU. Effects of message anxiety on disease detection and health promotion behaviors. *Basic Appl Soc Psycol*. 1996;18(1):61–74.
15. Leshner G, Bolls P, Thomas E. Scare' em or disgust' em: the effects of graphic health promotion messages. *Health Commun*. 2009;24(5):447–458.
16. Rogers EM. Diffusion of Innovations. 4th ed. New York, NY: Free Press; 2003.
17. Impicciatore P, Pandolfini C, Casella N, et al. Reliability of health information for the public on the World Wide Web: systematic survey of advice on managing fever in children at home. *BMJ*. 1997;314:1875–1879.
18. Griffiths KM, Christensen H. Quality of web based information on treatment of depression: cross sectional survey. *BMJ*. 2000; 321(7275):1511–1515.
19. Li L, Irvin E, Guzmán J, et al. Surfing for back pain patients: the nature and quality of back pain information on the Internet. *Spine*. 2001;26(5):545–557.
20. Mathur S, Shanti N, Brkaric M, et al. Surfing for scoliosis: the quality of information available on the Internet. *Spine*. 2005;30(23):2695–2700.
21. Evans MW, Perle SM, Ndetan H. Chiropractic wellness on the web: the content and quality of information related to wellness and primary prevention on the Internet. *Chiropr Man Therap*. 2011;19(1):4.
22. Beck RS, Daughtridge R, Sloane PD. Physician-patient communication in the primary care office: a systematic review. *J Am Board Fam Pract* 2002;15:25–38.
23. Brandt LJ. On the value of an old dress code in the new millennium. *Arch Intern Med*. 2003;163(11):1277–1281.
24. Rehman SU, Nietert PJ, Cope DW, et al. What to wear today? Effect of doctor's attire on the trust and confidence of patients. *Am J Med*. 2005;118(11):1279–1286.
25. Lill MM, Wilkinson TJ. Judging a book by its cover: descriptive survey of patients' preferences for doctors' appearance and mode of address. *BMJ*. 2005;331(7531):1524–1527.
26. du Pré A. Communicating about Health. 2nd ed. Boston, MA: McGraw–Hill; 2005:70–71.

CHAPTER 5

Consumer Health Information and Literacy

Karen Bulow

Technology has made health information more accessible to patients. Despite easier access, health literacy still remains low for several Americans. This chapter will explore the demographics and behaviors of health information seekers and some of the avenues for finding health information, specifically those found on the Internet. Evaluation methods are discussed to help discern the quality of the websites. Last, it will give some guidelines on how to lead patients to good health information while mentioning other influences on patients' health choices.

e-PATIENTS

In the current scenario, the World Wide Web has had a profound effect on helping patients find their own health care information, and patients are willing to explore this new access point. These proactive patients are known as e-patients. A study by the Pew Internet and American Life Project from 2009 found that the web is the third most popular resource for health information, after health professionals and friends and family, with 61% of Americans having looked online for health information.[1] Another study shows that although patients prefer to go to their doctors for health information (49.5%), the reality is that 48.6% first go to the web, whereas only 10% initially went to a health care provider.[2] From 2001 to 2007, the number of e-patients on the web increased by 38%, and a large majority of them have said that finding health information online has increased their knowledge on treating a condition or disease.[3]

The demographics of e-patients tend to fall roughly along the same lines as one would expect to see for general Internet users.[1] According to the Pew study, there are slightly more women than men seeking health information. In addition, this study has found that there are slightly more whites than African Americans, followed by Hispanics, and more educated and wealthier people tend to

go online more frequently. Younger adults are also more liable to seek online information and are also less likely to talk to a health professional. Those with less education tend to consult with a health professional less often than those with more education.[3] Of those that go online, a little over half are found to be searching on behalf of someone else.[1]

Sadly, about one-third of all Americans have low levels of health literacy.[4] Those with lower levels have a harder time following instructions for managing their health, let alone competently understanding their condition or disease.[4] Most of those with lower rates of literacy are those with less education. Minorities and immigrants tend to fall into this category as well.[5]

e-PATIENT SEARCHES

Table 5.1 describes the more popular health subjects that are researched by e-patients on the web. The categories in Table 5.1 have been tracked before in a previous Pew survey in 2002, and all of the categories have grown significantly in 7 years. One of the most significant growths in the search categories has been the number of adults seeking exercise or fitness information. It has grown from 21% to 38%, which is almost twice as much as reported in the 2002 survey.[1] Table 5.2 represents new categories to the survey that are also popular topics e-patients tend to research.

The information that e-patients find on the web seems to significantly affect many of their health care decisions. Sixty percent of information seekers say they know of someone who has benefited by the Internet health information, or they themselves have been helped by it.[1] The same percentage of e-patients have said that the information they found had some impact on decisions they made about their health, and about 13% of these online health searchers claim that the information had a major impact on them.[1] It

TABLE 5.1	Topics on Which Patients Seek Medical Information on the Web	
Topic		**Percentage**
A specific disease or medical problem		49
A medical treatment or procedure		41
Exercise or fitness information		38
Prescription or over-the-counter drugs		33
Alternative treatments or medicines		26
Depression, anxiety, stress, or mental health issues		21
Experimental treatments or medicines		15

Source: From Fox S, Jones S. *The Social Life of Health Information*. Washington, DC: Pew Internet & American Life Project;, 2009, with permission.

TABLE 5.2	Additional Topics on Which e-Patients Seek Information	
Topic		**Percentage**
Doctors or other health professionals		35
Hospitals or other medical facilities		28
Health insurance, including private insurance, Medicare, or Medicaid		27
How to lose weight or how to control your weight		24
How to stay healthy on a trip overseas		9

Source: From Fox S, Jones S. *The Social Life of Health Information*. Washington, DC: Pew Internet & American Life Project;, 2009, with permission.

is interesting to note that only 3% of e-patients knew of someone who had been harmed by online medical information. Table 5.3 contains some other statistics about how those searches impacted the e-patients

The third point in this table represents a significant phenomenon. It demonstrates that the information an e-patient finds spurs them on to seek professional advice in a little over half of adults. The survey did not take into account the quality of the information they found. Therefore,

TABLE 5.3	Impact of the Information e-Patients Find on the Web	
Topic		**Percentage**
The information found online affected a decision about how to treat an illness or condition		60
It changed their overall approach to maintaining their health or the health of someone they help take care of		56
It led them to ask a doctor new questions, or to get a second opinion from another doctor		53
It changed the way they think about diet, exercise, or stress management		49
It affected a decision about whether to see a doctor		38
It changed the way they cope with a chronic condition or manage pain		38

Source: From Fox S, Jones S. *The Social Life of Health Information*. Washington, DC: Pew Internet & American Life Project, 2009, with permission.

whether or not they found quality information, it still urged them to seek professional advice.

THE WORLD WIDE WEB

When a medical professional looks for information, they usually go to a trusted source, such as a professional database or a well-known medical journal, to find information on their subject of interest. How do they know that the information found in a professional database or journal is trustworthy? Health information for professionals tends to have some checks and balances in place to keep the quality of professional medical information relatively stable.

Owing to a lack of checks and balances for consumer health information, the web's health-related websites and databases are created with varying degrees of credibility.[6] Therefore, it can be hard for e-patients to know which ones to trust. It is difficult to get a good estimate of the percentage of poor health-related websites on the web because the percentage can vary with the subject matter and the person or persons analyzing the data. In general, regardless of the number of poor websites, there is good information out there if a person has the skills to find it.

A patient's ability to find quality health information on their own varies according to their level of health information literacy. The old Chinese proverb "Give a man a fish and feed him for a day. Teach a man to fish and feed him for a lifetime" is true for consumer information. Therefore, it is more important than ever to take the time to steer patients toward quality consumer information.

There are five points that the National Network of Libraries of Medicine (NN/LM) teaches to evaluate the trustworthiness of consumer information: Accuracy, authority, bias, coverage, and currency.[7] These five criteria do not focus on the functionality of a website, but on the trustworthiness of the information. These points tend to overlap each other frequently. One other criterion added in this chapter is design, which does address functionality. Although design does not reflect the content of the information, it does center on the user's needs for accessing and understanding the information. The steps are not written in alphabetical order below, but in the order that works best to establish a website's credibility.

Authority

When establishing authority, ask these questions:

- Who created this website?
- What are their credentials?
- For whom did they create this website?
- Whose money was used to create it?
- What proper names are listed on the website?
- Is the contact information legitimate?
- Is this a real person or business?
- Does this person have the right credentials or knowledge?
- Is this person enough of an authority on this subject to be trusted?

E-patients are not professionally trained in the practice of medicine. Due to their lack of having a professional medical education, they may have a hard time with some of the following evaluation points. Authority tends to be the easiest criterion to evaluate, and therefore it is a good place to start for evaluating a website.

There are many types of sources of health information on the web with varying degrees of authority. Some of these sources are associations, government agencies, hospitals, individuals, institutions, nonprofits, blogs, and product advertisers to name a few. All sources have their role to play in health literacy. None of them are considered truly bad or perfectly good.

Anyone with a vested interest and influence on the website can be considered an authority. Those presenting facts and opinions are authorities whether or not the website was created by them. Sometimes the authority is indirectly associated with the creation of the website. For example, Institution X awarded Nonprofit Y grant money to create a website promoting healthy eating. Institution X can be seen as an indirect authority. In such cases, try to pick up on the flow of money. This will help establish not only authority but also bias.

One way to test authority is to see whether legitimate contact information is provided on the website. If it is a hospital's website, find out whether the hospital is real by looking for their information on a couple of other websites. It is important to ensure that the names, addresses, and phone numbers on the website really exist and direct a person to the correct business. Closely examine the ways in which visitors to the website can contact the authority. The most trustworthy contact information is a real, physical address, not a post office box. Phone numbers are not quite as secure as a confirmation tool, but the worst contact points are e-mail addresses and contact forms that a person fills out online. These do not give enough information to ensure that the patient's information is going to the advertised authority. Unfortunately, more businesses are going to the contact form or e-mail model without realizing how it can hurt their authority.

Next, establish whether the person, business, or organization has the background to be an authoritative source for the patient's health information need. If an e-patient is looking for information on the outcomes of diabetic treatments, a highly authoritative source, such as the American Diabetes Association's (ADA) website, would be a very good choice. If that e-patient is trying to find out what it is like to live with diabetes, the ADA website probably has information on that, and an established doctor's opinion may be good, but so would a support group of people who live daily with the disease, although none of them may be a doctor. Authority only needs to be as authoritative as the search need establishes.

Currency

When establishing currency, ask these questions:

- How often is this website updated?
- Is there a copyright date, or any date on the website indicating its currency?
- What are the dates of its cited resources?
- Should it be updated more frequently due to the subject matter?

Currency is easily established when that information can be found. Some websites, however, will not give out this information. Many websites tend to have a copyright date or range on it, or they will advertise when the website was last updated. The *last updated* date is the most valuable to find. They give the most accurate understanding of the currency of the information. The copyright dates aren't quite as reliable. They may not reflect updates to the website since it was established, but they can indicate when a website was created or updated. Other dates that may be useful on websites are the dates on any cited books or articles, if any are given. If a website mentions other information sources (possibly in a bibliography), check the currency of those sources. Some new websites may cite very old information.

Owing to the fast pace of advances in medical information, e-patients should compare the currency of a website's information with their knowledge of the subject matter to establish whether the information is out of date. For example, it is usually fine to look at a 10-year-old website on anatomy, but it is usually not good to do the same for information on AIDS medication. This may be difficult for patients to do if they are not familiar with the advances in their subject matter.

Bias

When establishing bias, ask these questions:

- Does the website give all points of view on this topic?
- Does the website lean more toward one point of view than another?
- Does advertising play a role in influencing the opinions on this website?
- Is there any subtle product placement advertising?
- How many formal names can I spot?
- Is anyone trying to sell me something?
- Who endorses this website?
- Is this an opinion or a fact?

Bias comes in a variety of forms and can be both obvious and hard to find in consumer health information. Biased information is not necessarily wrong information. There may be a lot of good information on a biased website. The important thing is to recognize the biases and take them into consideration when forming a personal opinion of the information given.

The most prolific bias on the web is advertising. Advertising shows the flow of money and therefore demonstrates who is profiting from convincing readers to buy a product. If the website holds information that conflicts with the advertisement, that advertiser will most likely stop paying the site to advertise its products. For example, one would usually not see an advertisement from a major pharmaceutical company on a website for natural healing, but would not be surprised to see advertising of antidepressants on websites about depression. The depression advertisement creates a bias as it influences a patient to go to their doctor for a specific drug brand instead of a competitor's drug or talk therapy. Some websites are created strictly as advertising tools, and they are easy to spot by looking at the authority of the website. Although advertisements create bias, they don't usually give false information, though sometimes it may seem misleading.

Other biased information comes from more amateur websites created by one or perhaps a couple of individuals who just want to vent their biased views. These are usually pretty easy to spot as they are geared more toward someone's opinion than based on facts. When finding facts on sites like these, it is important to find the original source of the facts to establish that they are true.

There are some difficult types of bias to detect. For example, sometimes companies create "informational" websites on a specific condition or disease without marketing their company upfront. These companies are not just giving out health information for e-patients' benefits, but like every other company, they have a financial interest in arming e-patients with the information that they control. Go to a major search engine and search for information about weight loss. Look at the authorities involved in providing that information. Sometimes these websites say very little about the company, and play down their role in the creation of the website, but just a click or two of the mouse may send readers to more information about products that the company sells.

Other subtle biases tend to be more reputable, but still should be seen as a bias. For example, the American Chiropractic Association (ACA) will have great information on the benefits of manipulative therapy for spinal conditions, whereas the American Association of Orthopedic Surgeons (AAOS) will have great information on the benefits of surgery for the same conditions. Neither website is trying to be something other than what it is, but each shows different treatments for the same conditions. These sites will not present the other treatments as strongly as the ones they recommend.

The above examples are just some types of biases that e-patients may find on the web.

There are many more examples. The next topic is on two other potential types of bias: Accuracy and coverage.

Accuracy and Coverage

When establishing accuracy and coverage, ask these questions:

- How true is the content of this website?
- How does this website compare with others on the same topic?
- Do I know enough about this topic to be a good judge of the accuracy of this website?
- How much depth of coverage do I need?
- What parts of this subject are not fully covered?
- What are the underlying reasons to leave out this information?

Inaccurate information may be easy for the professional to spot, but it is not always that easy for the patient. How can a patient tell if they are reading inaccurate information? The short answer is they usually cannot. A person cannot know whether the information is wrong if they don't know it already. But if someone already knows the information they are seeking, then they wouldn't be researching it in the first place.

Coverage works similarly as accuracy. If a man walks into his living room, he can tell if something is missing. If that same man walked into someone else's living room, there's a good chance he won't notice if something is missing because he is not familiar with the room. Coverage of a health topic works the same way. It is almost impossible to know when something is missing unless one is already familiar with the subject.

Sometimes websites do not fully cover subjects to create bias in their favor. This of course also creates inaccurate information. Be sure not to confuse lack of depth with poor coverage. It is important to understand the degree of depth that is needed to answer the subject in question. One must first have a very clear understanding of what he or she is seeking to know— the amount of information needed and the depth of those answers.

Even though accuracy and coverage are difficult issues, there is a method that an e-patient or a health care provider can use to help them discern these criteria. This method should be seen by the e-patient as secondary to talking to a health care professional about the information they have found. To establish accuracy and/or coverage, find other websites that give the same information to verify the findings on the original website. This method is flawed, but it is usually the best an e-patient can do. These verification websites can come in two types.

The first type is verifying information with a website that has already been established as reputable. It should be a health-centered website that has given accurate and fully covered information in the past on health-related subjects. Health care providers are encouraged to use well-established and reputable professional databases and websites that also provide consumer information. Government-established websites like MedlinePlus tend to be safe bets. Websites of professional organizations or nonprofits are also well-established sources, though they may carry some legitimate bias. There are also several fee-based websites and databases from well-known publishers that could provide verification.

The second type of website an e-patient can visit is one that may not be as well established but meets the other four points of website evaluation. Looking at unfamiliar websites to verify information is not the safest route. But information on certain subjects is scarce, so sometimes taking any information that can be found is all that can be done. It is unfortunate, and can be very dangerous. Please use this method of verifying accuracy through unfamiliar websites with great caution. Not all websites cite their resources, so it is hard to know from where they got their information. If the verification website got their information from the original website, then of course the information will be the same. Look at a minimum of three websites to establish correct information.

The best way to smartly verify information with unfamiliar websites is to look for the ones that have won an award for giving good health information. Better yet, look up health information on these sites first. These awards are given by various groups. The most well-recognized one is the Health On the Net Foundation (HON) award. When looking for these awards on websites, ensure that they are legitimate awards and correctly posted to the website. Verify the awarded website with the website that gave them the award.

Design

When establishing good design, ask these questions:

- What are the physical and comprehension needs of this specific patient?
- Does this website accommodate their needs?
- Does this website write information at a level that matches my patient's level of understanding?
- Are there any cultural accommodations to make regarding images?

The design of a website may not always constitute a credible source, but it is an important consideration for many e-patients. Some of them may have visual problems and would prefer a website that accommodates their visual needs. Some of these visual needs may involve color choices for the color-blind or large text for those with poor eyesight. Those with carpal tunnel syndrome or arthritis may appreciate websites where minimal use of the mouse and keyboard are involved.

Besides physical issues, there are comprehension issues to take into consideration. Some e-patients may not be as savvy online and may have trouble understanding how to navigate the website. When they find information, the writing level may greatly impact the patient's ability to understand the information. Remember those with lower levels of health literacy need information that is written on a more basic level.

The visual impact of consumer information can play a key role for patients' understanding and recall of information, especially for those with lower health literacy, and the more pictures that enhance the health information, the better they will comprehend and remember it.[8] Don't forget to consider the effect of culture relative to the context of images. Some cultures may find certain pictures too graphic and may have a negative reaction toward the information.

RECOMMENDED RESOURCES

There are a couple of lists health professionals should be familiar with that cover good health information websites. The first is the Consumer and Patient Health Information Section (CAPHIS) Top 100 websites; http://caphis.mlanet.org/consumer/druginfo.html. This list is created by the Medical Library Association, and the list is categorized by subject. Another is the HON website; http://www.hon.ch. This is a well-recognized website that evaluates Internet health sources for quality information. On this website, a person can search for all the HON Code website awardees. Also recommended is MedlinePlus; http://www.nlm.nih.gov/medlineplus. This government website has information in several languages now, and it keeps adding more. This website links out to other quality sites on the web and also has a number of interactive videos to help facilitate the understanding of health conditions and procedures. The videos, in particular, are good for those with low levels of health literacy. Another quality government website is NIH SeniorHealth http://nihseniorhealth.gov. This website is made specifically for seniors who may have more trouble with vision and navigating websites. It is very user friendly and understandable for those with low health literacy.

Other Influences on e-Patients' Health Care Choices
SEARCH ENGINE RANKINGS

Many e-patients start at a search engine to find health care information.[9] Not many of them dig deep through the results of a search engine. Should this be a concern, or does all the good information rise to the top of these lists? Knowing how a search engine ranks websites will help patients understand how deep to look for information.

Not all websites are accessible through every search engine. A larger percentage of the more popular health information websites are usually in all the major engines, but understand that no search engine carries every health care website.

Be aware that there is no person looking through all the websites on the web, analyzing them for content and putting the best pages first. Algorithms are used to rank results on search engines. Each search engine uses its own blend of criteria to create their algorithm, but in general, they take several of the same factors into consideration when giving results. The first factor is the frequency of the searched word or phrase on a website's webpage, and also its frequency in the hidden content of the webpage, known as metadata. They also look at where that word or phrase is found on that webpage. The webpage is ranked higher if the word or phrase is found in the title of a webpage than if it is just a word used at the bottom of the webpage. Webpages with the most visitors and the highest number of other webpages linking to it rank higher in search engines.[10]

Some engines are starting to customize their results to their users. For example, Google ranks the websites a searcher has visited most often higher on the list of results.[11] They will also customize results by the searcher's location to help them get more local information.[12] Therefore, someone in New York who is constantly researching smoking cessation websites in Google will get very different results than someone in Alabama who is researching the same topic in Google for the first time.

DIRECT-TO-CONSUMER ADVERTISING

Direct-to-consumer advertising, also known as DTCA, has become much more prevalent in the past two decades.[13] Examples of DTCA can be found in newspapers, magazines, television, and of course, the web. DTCA has had a direct effect on the number of patients asking for prescription drugs.[14] One study noticed that 14% of patients in the Sacramento, California area requested prescription drugs due to DTCA.[15] Another study indicated that 50% of patients said they would be disappointed if their health care provider did not honor their prescription request, and another 15% of patients said they would consider switching doctors if they did not get the prescription drug they requested.[14]

Studies have shown that DTCA affects not only patients but also the prescribing patterns of health care providers. If a patient asks for a drug due to DTCA, 75% of the time their physician will prescribe that drug.[15] When requested by a patient, primary care physicians prescribe a drug 30% to 36% of the time when they would have prescribed the patient an alternative drug instead.[14] Many primary care physicians do see DTCA as poor influence on their patients owing to the bias and misleading information within the advertising.[16]

DTCA should not be seen solely as a negative influence, though. One study shows that a little over a quarter of patients they surveyed saw some form of DTCA that spurred them to ask their doctor for the first time about a condition or disease.[13]

TALKING TO THE e-PATIENT ABOUT HEALTH INFORMATION

When a health professional gives a patient information on their disease, they can control the quality of that information. When the patient finds that information for themselves, the patient now controls the quality of the information they receive. Therefore, it can be a great advantage for the health care provider to give out consumer information. When doing this, remember the characteristics of the patient that will influence the type of information that would best suit their needs. Take into consideration their literacy level and their native language. When working in an area with a large class of nonnative speakers, ensure that information can be provided in the dominant languages of the patient population. If there is little information in those languages, then obtain information in the most dominant secondary languages that caters to those with lower rates of literacy. It is also good to have on hand a list of credible websites with consumer information to steer patients in the right direction on the web.

With almost half of the population first seeking information online before going to a health professional, a significant number of e-patients are coming into their doctors' offices with preconceived notions of what they expect their doctors to do.[2,14] If a patient comes in armed with information, do not dismiss their efforts regardless of the quality of that information. The fact that they made this effort is a sign of their willingness to be responsible for their health. Remember there is a chance that the patient may feel the need to switch doctors if their efforts are not taken into consideration.[14] Instead, they should be complimented on their willingness to become active in their own health. There are some points to discuss when a patient comes in with health information. This may be a particularly delicate talk when the patient challenges a professional's health care decisions with consumer information.

There is a great clinical pearl originally written on a four-step process for managing cyberchondriacs, but the four steps can be enhanced to apply to any patient.[17] The first step is to assess the patient's competency. The paper originally meant a psychiatric competency, but for this purpose, it should include their health literacy level. Next, assess the information they present. Use the six steps mentioned above to guide them through the assessment. Then talk to the patient about the risks and benefits of acting on the information they found, and present the risks and benefits of other procedures that the professional feels should be considered.

When steering a patient toward a treatment other than the one they would prefer, first ensure that they understand how much you appreciate the effort they put into researching their condition. Then they should be informed that what works for one patient doesn't necessarily work for all, and that professional research and/or experience may steer the health care professional toward a different solution than what the patient may have found on their own. This does not mean that professionals should dismiss patient preferences, but it should be seen as one of several factors that should be weighed. Last, the patient and the professional should decide on a plan of action. Ultimately, finding common ground with the patient is integral for the patient's health and patient retention for the health care professional.

Health care professionals should try to be understanding of anxious patients. Patients get only one body, and it is the most personal object they own. Having other people tell them what they should do with their body when the person giving the orders doesn't have to live daily with the consequences of them, can be hard for an e-patient to accept if they expected a different treatment plan.

CONCLUSION

There are a lot of advantages to gathering health information on the web, and there are wonderful websites that can help e-patients make important decisions or support them in their health efforts. If in doubt about the quality of information, try to look for these types of information providers: government websites, well-known nonprofit associations, foundations, academies, trusted professional websites, hospitals, institutions of higher education, and award winning websites for health information. First, evaluate the authority of the information. Next, look at the currency of the information, and look at it in the context of the subject matter. Start reading the information while looking for biases, including advertisements and opinions. After reading, consider the accuracy and coverage of the information. Then check the information with other sources to verify it. Think of the patients and their ability to understand it. When patients wants to discuss the health information they found on their own, remember that they are showing both concern for their health and a willingness to play an active role by acquiring this information. Their efforts should be commended and the information they found should be discussed thoroughly.

Literature Cited

1. Fox S, Jones S. *The Social Life of Health Information*. Washington, DC: Pew Internet & American Life Project; 2009.
2. Hesse BW, Nelson DE, Kreps GL, et al. Trust and sources of health information: the impact of the Internet and its implications for health care providers: findings from the first Health Information National Trends Survey. *Arch Intern Med.* 2005;165(22):2618–2624.
3. Tu HT, Cohen GR. Striking jump in consumers seeking health care information. *Track Rep.* 2008;(20):1–8.
4. Riley JB, Cloonan P, Norton C. Low health literacy: a challenge to critical care. *Crit Care Nurs Q.* 2006;29(2):174–178.
5. Kutner MA. *The Health Literacy of America's Adults*. Washington, DC: U.S. Dept. of Education, National Center for Education Statistics; 2006.
6. Eysenbach G, Powell J, Kuss O, et al. Empirical studies assessing the quality of health information for consumers on the world wide web: a systematic review. *JAMA,* 2002;287(20):2691–2700.
7. Benedetti JA. From snake *oil to penicillin: Evaluating consumer h*ealth information on the inter net.http://nnlm.gov/training/consumer/snakeoil/. Accessed January 5, 2010.
8. Houts PS, Doak CC, Doak LG, et al. The role of pictures in improving health communication: a review of research on attention, comprehension, recall, and adherence. *Patient Educ Couns.* 2006;61(2):173–190.
9. Fox S. *Health Information Online*. Washington, DC: Pew Internet & American Life Project; 2005.
10. Staff S. How search engines rank web pages 2007. 1/05/12, http://searchenginewatch.com/article/2064539/How-Search-Engines-Rank-Web-Pages. 2011.
11. Horling B, Kulick M. Personalized search for everyone. The official Google blog. 2009., http://googleblog.blogspot.com/2010/10/this-week-in-search-102210.html#!/2010/10/this-week-in-search-102210.html
12. Singhal, A., This week in search 10/22/10, in The official Google blog. 2010, Google.
13. Lee AL. Changing effects of direct-to-consumer broadcast drug advertising information sources on prescription drug requests. *Health Commun.* 2009;24(4):361–376.
14. Lee AL. Who are the opinion leaders? The physicians, pharmacists, patients, and direct-to-consumer prescription drug advertising. *J Health Commun.* 2010;15(6):629–655.
15. Mintzes B, Barer ML, Kravitz RL, et al. How does direct-to-consumer advertising (DTCA) affect prescribing? A survey in primary care environments with and without legal DTCA. *CMAJ.* 2003;169(5):405–412.
16. Lipsky MS, Taylor CA. The opinions and experiences of family physicians regarding direct to consumer advertising. *J Fam Pract.* 1997;45(6):495–499.
17. Keller GL, Padala PR, Petty F. Clinical pearls to manage cyberchondriacs. *Prim Care Companion J Clin Psychiatry.* 2008;10(1):75–76.

CHAPTER 6

Advocating for Health in the Community

Marion W. Evans, Jr.

Advocacy is Latin for "voice." The *Directors of Health Promotion and Education* (DHPE) has defined advocacy as a step between educating people and lobbying for change.[1] Christoffel[2] defined it as the application of information and resources, which could include financial resources, efforts, or even votes, to effect systematic changes in a community.

Regardless of the definition, most people have a certain concept in mind when they hear the word that indicates one person or group is helping another for the greater good. Health promotion as a science is concerned with advocacy since it may involve not only educating people but also attempts to change health policy, laws, or even social norms. Advocacy within the greater community could be aimed at any or all of those when there is an interest in fostering better health in a community through positive social changes.

We have stated that micro issues within health and wellness include education and issues surrounding the individual, items inherent to an individual such as their personal genetic makeup, their family medical history, and knowledge or beliefs about a subject. Macro issues are those larger, social issues that must often be addressed at the community level.[3] The American Century Dictionary defines community as "a body of people living in one locale."[4] This can even include communities of workers at a plant or a college community. However, for the context of this chapter, the community is the area the reader lives and works in, and the issues are typically going to be at the macro level. Focusing on the macro level in addition to micro considerations, limits the tendency to blame the victim of a negative health situation because one must also examine the larger social view. Social standards, access to health services, policies, and regulatory agencies may all play a role in the health of a society; therefore, the notion that health is only an individual responsibility cannot serve as a successful model unless the larger ecological picture is taken into account. Epidemiological data also support a larger range of social issues that affect health, including a health care system that places too much reliance on individual behavior.[5]

ECOLOGICAL FRAMEWORK AND SYSTEMS THEORY

McLeroy and colleagues[6] outlined how an "ecological" framework can guide those in the field of health promotion and wellness in accounting for the various influencing factors on health status. This perspective suggests that only parts of the health paradigm occur under the influence and control, if you will, of the patient or individual. In this theoretical rubric, the person, their environment, and health behaviors are all interacting. Intrapersonal issues as discussed in Chapter 2 are those under the micro control of the individual, and they include knowledge, attitudes, or beliefs. Interpersonal relationships also play a role in that family, friends, coworkers, the family doctor, and others may influence the decisions of the individual. Under the macro umbrella are the larger, social items such as what happens in the community, including community norms, policies, and laws. Community norms may differ from one area or region of the country to another. What is accepted there? The standard level of knowledge or acceptable level of government involvement are issues that are considered macro issues, and those health professionals wanting to stress prevention, health promotion, and wellness measures should know what is most acceptable in their community beyond individual knowledge or control. Laws vary from one state to the next. Take, for example, motorcycle helmet laws; in some states they are required by all riders; in others, anyone over 21 can simply choose to ride without one. And institutions often have rules that make the grounds completely smoke free, whereas others may allow smoking on limited sections of the property. From these examples, it should be easy to see that there are multiple levels of influence related to health in the community.

Systems Theory

Systems theory simply suggests that there is a larger, overarching picture that we must view if we want to really see what is going on in a community or even an organization.[7] For example, most of us work within the "health care system." We may have an individual practice but we are part of a larger system, whether we want to believe it or not. Some practitioners may say, "I'm opting out of health insurance, and I'm only going to see patients for cash." Well, that is possible but in the case of Medicare, if you see the patient, you are subjected to rules, regulations, and coding requirements, and you will have to file the insurance for the patient or simply not see them at all. That's because Medicare requires doctors who treat Medicare-aged patients to be a part of the larger Medicare health care system. Systems theory suggests that no individual is acting alone but rather in a complex and dynamic environment where events are happening all around them that alter the ultimate outcome. In an advocacy role whereby the health care provider wants to influence community health, this must be kept in mind. Table 6.1 indicates some micro-level influences in the community along with factors that affect the community on a more macro level using the need for increased physical activity in America as an outcome of interest.

Typically, a combination of micro and macro approaches are needed to address community health issues. Individuals need to have the knowledge, the self-efficacy, and the personal motivation to change health behaviors. In addition, it is well recognized that these variables are not the same in all groups or communities and there may be a greater need to advocate for health resources. For example, if you have ever tried to walk down a busy street that has no sidewalks, you realize how unsafe and difficult it can be just to get from point A to point B. At times we ask our patients to increase their physical activity levels, but where will they do this if their street is poorly lighted, has no sidewalk, and is located in a busy part of town? This may provide an opportunity to approach a city council, county commission, philanthropy, or other group to come to the aid of the citizenry. Advising a patient to walk is a micro approach. Getting the city council to put in a walking path so he has a place to walk in his neighborhood is a macro approach. In an ecological framework, in a systems theory process, both may be necessary. Regardless of what one decides to advocate, at some point an opportunity to become involved at the community level may present itself. As a health care provider you are viewed as the expert in your community on health matters. Positively affecting the community is an often slow process that requires the 3Ps of advocacy: *Planning, patience,* and *partners.*

TABLE 6.1	Community Interactions at the Micro and Macro Levels Using Ecological Constructs
Level	**Action**
Intrapersonal	Educate patients and community leaders about the need for increased physical activity levels (increase knowledge and change personal attitudes)
Interpersonal	Work with community to form a walking club or stair-walking group at their office
Community	Sponsor local events that encourage walking and increased physical activity and health, such as the Komen Foundation Walk or Heart Association Walks
Policy	Work with local businesses and industries to establish wellness policies so that employees can be incentivized for increasing physical activity levels
Laws or community politics	Lobby for increased sidewalks, walk or bike paths, street lighting, where it may be unsafe to walk in the evenings without it

COMMUNITY NEEDS ASSESSMENT AND PLANNING

Before any community effort or advocacy opportunity, careful *planning* is essential. This first "P" is critical for success. Planning is probably best started with a *needs assessment*. The needs assessment is somewhat like a health care provider's workup of a patient. You look at the history with your patient, their family history, review of systems, vital signs, and so on. In a community, you will need to assess the history of the region. Where does the county or city rank in health within the region? Is it a low socioeconomic (SES) region without many resources, or is it an area of increasing wealth? Needs will vary according to SES levels. What is the ecological assessment of the area? What are the resources that *are* available? Is there a community center? If so, what does it have? Is there a YMCA, churches with facilities that could be used even to host a meeting of interested parties or a coalition? Planning should begin with looking at the current needs of your community. These should be actual needs that can assist you in reaching better health outcomes and not simply a wish list of items that some of your people would like to have. Separation of actual needs from perceived needs will take some patience. And that's the next "P."

Coalitions and Partners

Community processes, by nature, involve a lot of people. They may even involve city council members or others who don't really share your point of view. Developing a coalition of interested people who do share those interests will take time. Every effort should be made to include everyone who has an interest in this group. Sometimes, it even helps to have a few people on your coalition who may not completely agree with you. They will often tell you where your issues with opposing groups are going to be but may also be swayed to your side when they see you are open to suggestions and want to include them in this process. Be patient and take time to develop these networks.

The last "P" in this advocacy map is partners. Whom do you need on your side to make things happen? Usually there are potential program champions in your community who really like what you are proposing. A program champion is someone who is well known and respected in your community, and if he or she stands up and declares support for your cause, a number of people will join them

just because they support the idea. Think of who this champion can be *prior* to developing a coalition or starting the process of planning something new. Have them on board early and your job will become much easier. The writer crafted and passed the first smoking ordinance in his community in 1990 and modified it in 2000 to add strength to the ordinance with the help of a coalition. The mayor, who had not been a vocal supporter of the ordinance, recently experienced a cancer diagnosis in a family member, and once the coalition was formed and the issue was gaining interest, he became a strong program champion for strengthening the smoking ordinance in the town.[8] It is difficult to know where your champion may be, but if you look around, and if you do this early in your planning process, this strong, well-known advocate for your cause can start the process off with some significant momentum and can bring in allies quickly.

Working in Your Community

Checkoway[9] outlined the community participation process as planning, social action, needs assessment, and program implementation. This suggests that community action can democratize the political process and strengthen leadership in a region. An example of a community need is the smoking ordinance mentioned earlier, which would restrict smoking to protect local citizens from environmental tobacco smoke. There are other local laws or ordinances that may fall into the same category such as laws that ban cell phone use in cars, impose teen curfews, add bike paths in a community, or even set up a skateboard park. Promoting the need for physical activity and after-school sports programs are other ideas that could be defined as needs in many communities. In many parts of the United States where obesity is becoming the norm rather than the exception, any program that stresses the need for increased exercise levels will be seen as a serious possible action to take. Providing places where physical activity can take place is a worthy goal to adopt in a society battling an obesity epidemic.

Once an actual need in the community is identified, the first step may be to contact a policy maker about the problem. Today this is often done by phone, letter, and even e-mail. Galer-Unti and colleagues[10] suggested the best strategy is meeting with your political representatives face-to-face. This could be a council member, statesman, or US congressman or congresswoman. You want to establish an ongoing personal relationship with them and it always helps to have a face with the name. One should remember that most political representatives at the local or even national level are typically not health care providers, so there is usually a need to educate them on the topic of health and social norms along with needed law or policy changes and why they should help your efforts. Educate them about the needs within the community. One should research the topic so they may provide the representative with details that make it easier to support the favored position. Checkoway[9] further stated the importance of recognizing that there may be unanswered questions and stressed the need for community participation when advocating a health promotion position. There will always be a need for buy-in from the community on a wholesale basis for the greatest chance of success. It should be noted here that federal aid can be found for local, community projects. Don't rule out help for your community at any level.

In addition to public policy, there may be opportunities to work within the community to establish community norms that are more conducive to health that are already ongoing. Support of entities outside of government that promote healthy activities and health promoting programs is also worthy of consideration. The *Komen Foundation* for breast cancer awareness and the *American Heart Association* (AHA) both have regional activities that support healthy behaviors in schools such as *Jump Rope for Heart*. Some health care providers may want to partner with the *Red Cross* to offer their building or parking lot as a site for delivery of *Red Cross* services on certain days of the month or host a blood drive. Certainly there are other health care providers worthy of support, but these are common in most communities and provide the examples of programs offering a chance to support health-oriented campaigns. This is an opportunity to form partnerships. Take advantage of this whenever possible.

Coalitions

The *Prevention Institute* established a "Spectrum of Prevention" for developing an effective coalition within the community.[11] This included influencing policy and legislation; changing organizational practices; fostering coalitions and networks; educating providers; promoting community education; and strengthening individual knowledge and skills. Taking this model upward from the base, one would first concentrate on individual knowledge and skill enhancement. Knowledge is necessary for positive behavior change but in

reality, is not enough. Education within the community is critical to build community awareness. And while education of various providers of services is also important, the *Prevention Institute* conceded that ecological/environmental support for healthy behavior typically comes from changing organizational practices or influencing policy and legislation. This often requires coalitions and networks within a community to accomplish.

Specific Community Approaches

Loue[12] suggested two major considerations related to advocacy within a community: (1) Grassroots or "bottom-up" approaches, where the needs are determined by community groups themselves, and (2) "Top-down" models, where needs are identified by outside experts or only by the leaders within a community. Both these models can be successful but it is also important to know that there can be guidance from outside experts that assists the community members in reaching their overall goals. This is where you can be of assistance in the process, thereby increasing the chances of their success.

When outside experts are involved, it is important to realize that if community partners or members do not feel involved in the decision-making process, the chance of success decreases. Once a need is defined for a community and the decision is made to advocate change with a coalition, some important considerations must be taken into account early in the planning stages. Will the members of the coalition be from the community or government groups or both? If the community is going to be involved, will the coalition take on anyone as a member? Make every effort to be all-inclusive wherever possible. It is probably a good idea to allow anyone to participate as long as they are supportive of the process. There must be organization to the efforts but allowing all interested parties to participate will create community-level buy-in. Cohen, Baer, and Satterwhite,[13] in their Eight Step Guide to effective coalitions (*Prevention Institute*), list these steps in the development of coalitions:

Step 1—Analyze the program's objectives and determine whether to form a coalition in the first place.

Step 2—Recruit the right people.

Step 3—Devise a set of preliminary objectives and activities.

Step 4—Convene the coalition.

Step 5—Anticipate the necessary resources.

Step 6—Define elements of a successful coalition structure.

Step 7—Maintain coalition vitality.

Step 8—Make improvements through evaluation.

Included in the above process is recruiting the key people in your community that get things done plus the local experts people will respect. They may not be health experts but if they are seen as trustworthy in the community they need to be involved in this process. Know your objectives up front. What if you hit a roadblock? Will you be open to a compromise if you can't get exactly what you originally set out for? You may want to discuss a fallback position early in the planning stages so everyone knows where the group stands on compromise. Remember, this is often the reality of a political process, as there will usually be multiple interest groups involved anytime a change is proposed. Also, what resources will you need? Do you need money, manpower, editorial space from the local paper, TV coverage, a good blogger on your team? The process of community change, and particularly changes in local policies or laws, will likely take time. Be prepared to keep your coalition going, and keep your message alive and well in front of the public. Make necessary adjustments along the course. Nothing says you have to finish exactly as you started. Stay focused on the long-term goals and on how your efforts will improve the health of the community through successful changes in the status quo, and stay the course!

Program Champions

Every community has individuals who are known to get things done. Find one if you can. Who is the most influential in your community and likely to support your plan? Once you find one, educate him or her early in the process. Be clear and concise about what you want to accomplish and why. Frame it for what it is—a health issue. Provide them with support literature and information to make their decision an easy one and worthy of support. If you are aiming for a champion from the local government, take a council member's constituent base with you if you are going to meet them when this is possible. Just a couple can be effective at the initial level of discussion. Voters from the district can bring the issue home. This could sway them to become a champion of your cause all by itself. It doesn't hurt to stack the deck with constituents of the council member or commissioner, even if they are a champion, just to show that he or she has voters there supporting the effort once the topic is in the public forum. Should there be people in an audience who do not favor what you want to do, make it easy on your champion to point toward a full room of his supporters to rationalize why he is on board.

In some cases, preparing talking points or bullet points for your program champion may be helpful. If your champion is on the council or commission, help them educate their fellow board members. Ask them what form they prefer this material to be in. Again, it's about making their job easier to help you. If you are coming before a political group or policy making body, let them know up front you are coming and why. Get on their agenda so they are aware you will be coming. It doesn't hurt to provide information that supports your position at that time. Some city councils and county commissions have a 5-minute agenda where anyone who calls ahead can be placed on the speaking list for 5 minutes. Prepare remarks up front and have a few key speakers for your coalition lined up with talking points in hand. Stick to your message as planned! Leave them information that supports what you said behind to review in case they meet in sub-committees to discuss what you are asking for. And remember, this is a process that will take some time. Prepare to go before the decision-making body more than once and remind them you want to be present when your topic is being discussed, if possible. If you have a champion on the council or committee, ask them to have their office keep you informed or ask whom you can call in their office to stay abreast of changes in your item of interest. Some will have a health liaison in larger councils, county commissions, or in a statehouse or the US Congress. Keep your local media involved and appoint a spokesperson to deal with them from your coalition if this is needed. When the local media supports your efforts, it can keep your issues front-page news.

SUPPORT MATERIALS, TALKING POINTS, AND MEDIA PACKETS

In any event where you approach a city council, senator, school board president, or potential change agent, you may want to prepare a packet of materials for them that supports what you will say. These can be designed for the media as well. If you can identify the media person in charge of covering the legislative body you are lobbying, it may be a good idea to meet with him or her in advance and explain what you hope to accomplish. What you provide the council or legislative body can also support your position with the media. Media will often use exactly what you provide them so as to not have to do research on the topic themselves. Some will want to verify what you have told them, so you may want to include recent journal articles and articles from the newspaper or your favorite online source in the packet so they can see what you are using to make your point. It might also be appropriate to mention any specific, new information generated from your needs assessment that is unique to your community.

Support Materials

Generally, support materials should be short, to the point, and written on a fifth-grade level. Remember, these people you are likely convincing to take up your cause are probably not rocket scientists or health scientists. If you have ever spoken to a member of your statehouse, you get the idea. And you can always provide stronger, more sophisticated materials upon request. Think about using a folder with two pockets where you can outline your goals on one side on perhaps a Word document with your plan, plus a few bullet points. On the opposing side, add your support documents. Make sure you have a contact person should there be questions after you leave. This goes for the council or body you are speaking to and the media. These "leave-behind" materials should help make your point, so choose carefully what you provide them with. Within Microsoft Word on the spell-check feature you can add a "reading level" assessment feature from the tools menu. This will analyze anything you prepare in Word and tell you the grade reading level. We recommend no higher than a fifth-grade level for any health-related information. This is the approximate reading level of the average American, so keep it simple to avoid misunderstandings and get the message across effectively. A general rule of thumb is the more polysyllabic words, the higher the reading level. Having materials printed in color helps. Materials from recognized agencies such as your state health department, the Centers for Disease Control and Prevention (CDC), or the National Cancer Institute (NCI) because they are authoritative in nature. Most people don't question them, because they are considered a reputable source of information. Support material may also include websites that you would recommend for further reading on the topic.

Talking Points

So you have made it to the city council, you are on the 5-minute agenda, and are speaking for your new coalition. What are you going to say? It should be easy. Remember, you have framed all of this out in advance, planned, have been patient, you have your strategy, the rails are greased, and a program champion is in the room. Don't blow it now! Talking points need to relay the simple message you want them to hear. You may want to have five bullet points but probably not more than that. That only gives you a minute to cover each one, so if you can, make it fewer than 5 or list 5 quick points that don't take a lot of time to mention. And don't go to a councilman or any other politician thinking you are going to give them a mini-seminar. They will be discussing multiple agenda items that day and you will be one of them. You want to stand out but not because you were so long-winded they had to cut you off. Respect their time and the process, and prepare them by providing background information in advance and with the leave-behind materials you have carefully selected. And it is OK to follow up with an additional piece of information here and there to keep your cause in front of them until what you have advocated is a reality.

Media Packets

The media packet is aimed at providing the media with a background level of information on who you are, what you are asking for, support material that helps explain why you want change, whom it affects, and so on. In addition, you will want to provide the following:

- The name and proper pronunciation (if needed) of the key spokesperson for your group
- The contact information on how you want them to reach you if they need information or clarification, or want to interview you on the subject
- Times when you are available
- A time line to accomplish what you are advocating
- Key partners in your venture that they could contact to verify support of your cause (such as a program champion, if that person has agreed in advance to serve in this capacity)

Although you will likely explain what you want and why, it is a good idea to give media outlets any city, county, state, or national support data that you can that explain why you want changes made. Table 6.2 lists some excellent sources of data and health statistics that you may want to use in a

TABLE 6.2	Resources for Community Advocacy Groups	
Agency	**Resource**	**Website**
U.S. Census 2010 interactive population map	Shows population down to city or region of the city level	http://2010.census.gov/2010census/popmap
F as in fat: How obesity threatens America's future–2010	Stats on obesity and overweight problems in America, state-by-state scores, and possible interventions	http://healthyamericans.org/reports/obesity2010
America's Health Rankings	Stats on state-by-state rankings related to a variety of health risks	http://www.americashealthrankings.org/Rankings
County Health Rankings & Roadmaps	County stats on various health issues from the US	http://www.countyhealthrankings.org
U.S. Centers for Disease Control and Prevention	Numerous sites for health-risk data, information on prevention, screening, disease management, and Center for Health Statistics	www.cdc.gov
National Cancer Institute	Information on cancer stats and prevention of cancer through lifestyle changes	www.cancer.gov
Coalitions and Public Health (Prevention Institute)	Eight-Step Guide to coalition building	http://www.preventioninstitute.org/index.php?option=com_jlibrary&view=article&id=104&Itemid=127
Community Tool Box-University of Kansas	Information, tools for community health	http://ctb.ku.edu/en/default.aspx

community advocacy campaign. This is information that may likely come from the needs assessment.

HEALTH PROMOTION, ADVOCACY, AND PREVENTION OF SPORTS-RELATED INJURY

Williams and colleagues[14] outlined an advocacy opportunity for the health care provider to act as a community advocate related to prevention of injuries in recreational sports. Using an Ecological Framework at the intrapersonal level, they suggested the clinician could educate young athletes about injury prevention by teaching proper stretching techniques and warm-up routines along with proper sport nutrition, equipment safety, or taping. At the interpersonal level, relationships with other groups are suggested that include teaching coaches, staff, or athletic trainers about awareness or evaluation of injury. The authors used the CDC program "Heads-up," aimed at reducing concussion injury as an example.

At the institutional level, this example for injury prevention stressed that schools could be lobbied or educated about adoption of safe play rules such as not pressurizing an injured player to stay in the game. This could also be stressed at the recreational level. In the community, injury prevention messages, on-the-field injury prevention clinics, and volunteering as a medical provider or team doctors were stressed. Williams and colleagues concluded with the policy level and as an example suggested that clinicians could lobby schools to limit the availability of sport drinks that contain stimulants or questionable sport supplements in student athletes. While these are examples where advocacy can be used to promote health and safety, Figure 6.1 is an example of health advocacy in reverse. Motorcyclists have been successful in repealing helmet laws in many states through concerted advocacy efforts.

From the above example it should be easy to see that advocacy can be a part of several ventures in the community when it comes to changing health outcomes. This does not have to be aimed

Motorcycle helmet laws were enacted to save lives in cases of motorcycle crashes. Most states adopted these laws to protect riders from head injuries, which are often fatal. In spite of lower rates of fatal crashes in the 1980s and 1990s, advocates for the repeal of these laws appeared at various state legislatures in the name of freedom to ride and enjoy the open road. These motorcycle rider groups challenged the laws, suggesting that it should be their prerogative to take an increased risk if they wanted to do so.

As a result of lobbying efforts by various groups, states like Florida, Texas, and Pennsylvania (as well as others) repealed these safe riding laws regarding helmet use. Until April 2008, only 20 states mandated helmet use for all riders. The results have been startling. For example, in Florida, where prior to the repeal all riders had to wear a helmet (up to the year 2000), by the end of that year, motorcyclist fatalities had increased 45.5%. However, these laws are credited for having also increased sales and the number of riders.

After a 2003 repeal of the helmet law in Pennsylvania, head-related injury deaths increased 66%. Between 2002 and 2005, helmet use among riders in crashes decreased from 82% to 58%. The use of helmets has been estimated to reduce the risk of death by 42% and head injury by 69%; yet, advocates for the repeal of these laws have been successful in many states.

This example shows us that even advocacy for something that can increase risks can be accomplished if an effective plan is executed.

Figure 6.1. Health advocacy in reverse—The repeal of motorcycle helmet laws. (From Muller A. Florida's motorcycle helmet law repeal and fetality rates. Am J Public Health. 2004;94(4):556–558.)

only at changes in laws or government policy. At times it may be as simple as volunteering one's time to help promote safer play or voicing an expert medical opinion related to the need for a safer playground.

Literature Cited

1. Directors of Health Promotion and Education. *Lobbying and The Law: a Primer for Public Health Professionals*. Washington, DC: Directors of Health Promotion and Education; 2007:5.
2. Christoffel KK. Public health advocacy: process and product. *Am J Public Health*. 2000; 90(5): 722–726.
3. O'Rourke T. Philosophical Reflections on Health Education and Health Promotion: Shifting Sands and Ebbing Tides. *The Health Education Monograph Series*. 2006; 23(1):7–10.
4. *American Century Dictionary*. New York, NY: Oxford University Press; 1995:116.
5. Mu L, Shroff F, Dharamsi S. Inspiring health advocacy in family medicine: a qualitative study. *Educ Health (Abingdon)*. 2011; 24(1): 534.
6. McLeroy KR, Bibeau D, Steckler A, et al. An ecological perspective on health promotion programs. *Health Educ Q*. 1988; 15(4): 351–377.
7. Schultz JS. *Family Systems Therapy: an Integration*. Northvale, NJ: Aronson; 1984.
8. Evans MW Jr. Modification of a local smoking ordinance: a case-report of chiropractic health advocacy. *J Chiropr Med*.2006; 5(1): 32–37.
9. Checkoway B. Community participation for health promotion: prescription for public policy. *Wellness Perspectives: Research, Theory and Practice*. 1989; 6(1):18–26.
10. Galer-Unti RA, Tappe MK, Lachenmayr S. Advocacy 101: Getting Started in Health Education Advocacy. *Health Promot Pract*. 2004; 5(3):280–288.
11. Prevention Institute *Developing Effective Coalitions: An Eight Step Guide*. Oakland, CA: Prevention Institute; 2002.
12. Loue S. Community health advocacy. *J Epidemiol Community Health*. 2006;60(6):458–463.
13. Cohen L, Baer N, Satterwhite P. Developing effective coalitions: An eight step guide. In: Wurzbach ME, ed. *Community Health Education & Promotion:A Guide to Program Design and Evaluation*. 2nd ed. Gathersburg, MD: Aspen Publishers Inc.; 2002
14. Williams RD, Jr., Evans MW Jr., Perko MA. Health Promotion Advocacy: A Practitioner's Role in Prevention of Sports Injuries. *Topics in Integrative Health Care*. 2011; 2(1).2.1003.

CHAPTER 7

Wellness Assessment and Clinical Preventive Services

Cheryl Hawk

According to the U.S. Preventive Services Task Force (USPSTF), clinical preventive services as provided by medical physicians consist of screening, health behavior counseling, and immunizations and chemoprophylaxis.[1] For complementary and alternative medicine (CAM) practitioners providing manual therapies and other CAM procedures, but not medications or immunizations, we suggest a wellness model of care that includes manual procedures to optimize function, screening for risk factors, and health behavior counseling. These models have both screening and health behavior counseling in common. Many types of screening tests can be performed or ordered by various CAM practitioners, and the others can be referred out to medical physicians with whom the clinician has a collaborative and/or collegial relationship. Health behavior counseling is within the scope of practice of most CAM providers. To provide optimal wellness care, clinicians need to provide the most up-to-date, evidence-based screening and counseling, or, if these are not within their scope of practice, be able to make appropriate referrals for these. The USPSTF (http://www.ahrq.gov/CLINIC/uspstfix.htm) is the best source of current recommendations, and these are detailed in this chapter.

Clinical preventive services are recognized billable services for practitioners with the appropriate scope. In 1992, the American Medical Association (AMA), the body developing and trademarking the Current Procedural Terminology (CPT) codes, established a set of codes for Preventive Medicine Services (PMS) and Preventive Medicine Counseling (PMC). In 2008, smoking cessation counseling, both group and individual, was added to the PMC codes. Details on the PMS and PMC codes are available in the AMA CPT manual.[2] They are also explained in Chapter 23 of Woolf's Health Promotion and Disease Prevention in Clinical Practice, second edition.[3]

CPT publications, commonly used by chiropractors and other CAM providers whose scope of practice allows it, often do not include the codes for preventive services, so it isimportant to consult the AMA CPT manual.[2] If a patient's insurance plan does not cover PMS and PMC, the patient can be billed, if appropriate; however, it is important to be sure that the patient understands all the fees and the ones he or she will need to pay out of pocket.

PREVENTIVE SERVICES

Although certainly all patients, whether presenting for treatment or for wellness care, need risk factor identification and advice on prevention and health promotion, patients for whom preventive service codes are applicable are those with no complaint or current illness when they present for these services. The preventive services include complete history, examination, and screening and identification of risk factors. An essential point is that these services are age and gender specific, so it is necessary that the clinician be familiar with all age-specific risk factors and know how to identify them. This chapter describes these risk factors and provides resources for helping patients to reduce or eliminate them.

Specific codes for tobacco cessation counseling were added in 2008, for both individual and group counseling. See the AMA CPT manual for details.[2] Tobacco cessation counseling is one of the most important preventive services, because of the extremely high impact tobacco use has on the health of the public and on health care spending.

Wellness Assessment

Most patients present for treatment of symptoms or a condition. However, this also presents an opportunity to assist them in becoming aware of how they can improve their health and enhance or begin their wellness journey. Just as treatment begins with diagnosis and assessment, wellness care/health promotion begins with risk factor identification and lifestyle assessment. Table 7.1 summarizes these and refers to tools for measuring each parameter.[1] It should be remembered that wellness-based assessment takes place simultaneously with illness-based assessment, at the patient's first visit, with follow-up assessments at intervals appropriate for the parameters being measured (Tables 7.2 and 7.3; Figs. 7.1–7.3).

Clinical Preventive Services by Age Group

As indicated in Table 7.1, risk factor identification and counseling are age-specific. Information on the risk factor identification and counseling interventions recommended for each age group by the USPSTF are described in this chapter.[1]

Table 7.4 provides an overview for all the age groups, based on recommendations of the USPSTF. The specific practices and procedures appropriate for each age group are detailed in the following sections of this chapter.

TABLE 7.1	Multifactorial Wellness Screening and Assessment

Screening

Risk factors for disease, including but not limited to:

Blood pressure
Overweight/obesity (BMI: http://www.nhlbisupport.com/bmi/bmicalc.htm; calculator: see Fig. 6.1)
Tobacco use (former and current; see Table 6.2)
Physical activity (Table 6.3)
Diet (see Fig. 6.2)
Screen for other age-specific risk factors (Tables 6.9–6.11)

Depression (see Depression Screener text box)

Stress (see Perceived Stress Scale, Fig. 6.3)

Assessment

General health status (see BRFSS health status question, text box)

Well-being or vitality (see BRFSS energy question text box and GWBS, Fig. 6.4)

TABLE 7.2	Tobacco Use Screener Assessing Readiness to Quit

Do you currently smoke or use other tobacco products?

❏ Never ❏ Formerly, not now
❏ Yes, currently

If "yes," how interested are you right now in quitting or discussing how to quit?

❏ I'm not interested in quitting right now.
❏ I'm not able to quit right now.
❏ I'm thinking about quitting in the next 6 months.
❏ I'm planning to quit in the next month.
❏ I'm in the process of quitting right now.

❏ *Would you like to talk with the doctor about quitting?*

TABLE 7.3	Physical Activity Screening

Do you take part in either of the following?

❏ At least 2½ **total hours** (150 min) of moderate-intensity activity per wk. (Add up all sessions that are at least 10 min in duration)

Moderate means you are exercising at a level where you can talk, but not sing, such as brisk walking or lawn mowing.

OR

❏ At least **75 total minutes** (1¼ h) of vigorous-intensity activity per wk. (Add up all sessions that are at least 10 min in duration)

Vigorous means you are exercising at a level where you can say only a few words without pausing for breath, such as jogging/running, fast bike-riding.

Scoring: If neither box is checked, the patient is not getting the recommended amount of physical activity.

	Weight in Pounds		
Height	Normal	Overweight	Obese
5' 0"	95-127	128-153	154+
5'1"	97-132	133-158	159+
5'2"	101-136	137-163	164+
5'3"	105-140	141-169	170+
5'4"	108-145	146-173	174+
5'5"	111-149	150-179	180+
5'6"	115-154	155-185	186+
5'7"	118-159	160-191	192+
5'8"	122-164	165-196	197+
5'9"	125-168	169-202	203+
5'10"	129-173	174-208	209+
5'11"	133-178	179-214	215+
6'0"	137-183	184-220	221+
6'1"	140-189	190-227	228+
6'2"	144-194	195-233	234+
6'3"	148-199	200-239	240+
6'4"	152-204	205-246	247+

Figure 7.1. Overweight and obesity calculator.

OFFICE USE ONLY
Patient ID: _____
Score:_____Date:___/___/___

Nutrition Screening

1. Using the information about servings in this box, how many servings of fruits and vegetables do you usually eat daily?
   ① 0
   ② 1–2
   ③ 3–4
   ④ 5 or more

   Fruits and Vegetables:
   What is 1 serving?
   • 1 cup raw
   • ½ cup cooked
   • 1 medium fruit
   • ¾ cup (6 oz) juice (100% juice)

2. How often do you **SKIP** breakfast?
   ① Daily (that is, I never eat breakfast)
   ② Often skip it (several times a week)
   ③ Occasionally skip it
   ④ Never or rarely skip it

3. How often do you eat fast food (McDonald's, Burger King, etc)?
   ① Daily
   ② Often (several times a week)
   ③ Occasionally
   ④ Never or rarely

4. How often do you eat white bread or pasta?
   ① Daily
   ② Often (several times a week)
   ③ Occasionally
   ④ Never or rarely (I avoid bread and pasta OR I only use the whole grain type)

5. How often do you eat sweets and desserts?
   ① Daily
   ② Often (several times a week)
   ③ Occasionally
   ④ Never or rarely

6. How many 8-oz cups of soda (cola, 7-up, etc) do you drink **DAILY**? (one can is usually 12 oz, which equals 1 ½ cups)
   _____ cups per day, regular sweetener (sugar/sucrose)
   _____ cups per day, artificial sweetener (Nutrasweet, Splenda, etc)

7. Do you have any of the following special dietary needs/practices?
   ❒ Vegan
   ❒ Food allergies/sensitivities (like gluten intolerance)
   ❒ Weight-loss diet currently or last 6 months
   ❒ Other: _____

Figure 7.2. Nutrition screening questionnaire.

Scoring

Questions 1–5, score 1–4 points as indicated.
Question 6:
        0 cups = 4 points
        Any other amount = 0 points

Question 7:
        No dietary restrictions (no boxes checked) = 4 points
        Any boxes checked = 0 points

Interpretation

28 is the maximum possible score, 5 is the minimum possible.
A score < 15 indicates a need for additional dietary assessment.

Figure 7.2. *Continued*

Global Well-Being Scale

OFFICE USE ONLY
Pt ID: _____ Date: __ __/__ __/ 20__

Please think about how you are feeling right now--your general sense of health and well-being. On the line below, make a straight vertical (up-and-down) mark on the line to show how you feel right now.

WORST YOU COULD   _____   BEST YOU COULD
POSSIBLY FEEL   POSSIBLY FEEL

Figure 7.3. Global well-being scale.

Depression Screener

Over the past 2 weeks, have you ever felt down, depressed, or hopeless?

Over the past 2 weeks, have you felt little interest or pleasure in doing things?

An answer of "yes" to either question indicates a need for further assessment of possible presence of depression.

Source: USPSTF

Assessment of Well-Being/Energy

During the past 30 days, for about how many days did you feel very healthy and full of energy?

Source: Behavioral Risk Factor Surveillance Survey of the CDC

TABLE 7.4	Screening and Counseling by Age Group	
Age (y)	**Screening Tests/Risk Factor Identification**	**Counseling—For All Parents and Children**

0–1	Hearing
	Height and weight
	Head circumference
		Counseling for All Children
		  Development
		  Nutrition
		  Physical activity
		  Safety/injuries/poisoning
		  Violence/firearms

1–4	Height and weight Vision (3–4 y)	
5–11	Height and weight	**Additional Counseling for Teens**
12–17	Height and weight Major depressive disorder	STDs, HIV

18–39	**Screening Tests**
	
	  Blood pressure at least every 2 y
	  Cholesterol for men aged 18–35 y at risk, and women at risk
	  Diabetes for men and women at risk for heart disease
	  Cervical cancer for women (every 3 y)
	  BMI for obesity	

	Risk Factor Identification (Ask Patient)
	
	  Diet for men and women with high cholesterol or at risk for heart disease and diabetes
	  Tobacco use
	  Alcohol misuse
	  Depression	

40–64	**Screening Tests**
	
	  Blood pressure at least every 2 y
	  Cholesterol for all men and for women at risk up to age 45 y, all women over 45 y
	  Diabetes for men and women at risk for heart disease
	  Colorectal cancer—For men and women aged 50+
	  Cervical cancer for women (every 3 y)
	  Breast cancer for women (every 2 y starting at age 50 y)
	  BMI for obesity
	  Osteoporosis screening for women aged 60+ at risk	

	Risk Factor Identification (Ask Patient)
	
	  Diet for men and women with high cholesterol or at risk for heart disease and diabetes
	  Tobacco use
	  Alcohol misuse
	  Depression	

65 +	**Screening Tests**
	
	  Blood pressure at least every 2 y
	  Cholesterol for all men and women at risk
	  Diabetes for men and women at risk for heart disease
	  Breast cancer for women (every 1–2 y up to age 75 y)
	  Aortic aneurysm for men 65–75 y who have ever smoked
	  Colorectal cancer
	  BMI for obesity
	  Osteoporosis screening for women (2 y or > intervals)	

(*continued*)

TABLE 7.4	Screening and Counseling by Age Group (*continued*)	
Age (y)	**Screening Tests/Risk Factor Identification**	**Counseling—For All Parents and Children**
	Risk Factor Identification Diet for men and women with high cholesterol or at risk for heart disease and diabetes Tobacco use Alcohol abuse Depression	

Note: The USPSTF refers to the CDC for schedules for immunizations. The CDC provides these at: http://www.cdc.gov/vaccines/recs/schedules/pocketsize.htm
BMI, body mass index; STD, sexually transmitted disease.
Source: From USPSTF. Guide to Clinical Preventive Services, 2009: http://www.ahrq.gov/ppip/timelinead.pdf, with permission.

PREVENTIVE SERVICES—INFANTS (UP TO 12 MONTHS)

Example

An established patient brings her healthy, asymptomatic 3-month-old boy in for a well-baby checkup, including a general health evaluation. The clinician takes a complete history and performs a comprehensive physical examination with review of systems. The baby's growth and development are evaluated, including height, weight, head circumference, hearing, and developmental milestones. The clinician provides advice to the mother on correct use of the infant car seat; proper nutrition, emphasizing continued breast-feeding; and sleep practices. The clinician explains age-specific risk factors for injury and illness, along with methods to reduce or eliminate them.

Well-baby visits are an established part of good health care.[4] Clinicians who are experienced with working with infants and whose scope of practice allows them to assess their health status and health history should also advise parents on healthy nutrition, safety/injury prevention, and other lifestyle factors. Immunizations, a mainstay of medical preventive services, are not within the scope of practice of most CAM providers, so parents should be referred to their family medical physician on this topic. However, the Chiropractic Health Care Section of the American Public Health Association (APHA) maintains a website with evidence-based information on immunizations, so that doctors of chiropractic (DCs) and other CAM providers have ready access to current evidence, should parents ask them for information.[4,5]

Table 7.5 summarizes the recommendations made by the USPSTF on appropriate screening and counseling for infants.

For infants, recommended screening consists of hearing tests and assessment of height, weight, head circumference, and developmental milestones.

For counseling parents of infants, it is particularly important to emphasize the importance of breast-feeding and to provide parents with information on how to be successful at breast-feeding. The CDC manual listed in Table 7.5 gives providers ample evidence-based information to equip him or her to counsel patients on this important part of infant care. Counseling on injury prevention, both of unintentional and intentional injuries, is also essential. This includes instructions on proper sleep positions, since stomach-sleeping has been associated with Sudden Infant Death Syndrome (SIDS), the leading cause of death in infants in the United States. It has been found that physician advice is a significant factor in parents placing their infants on their backs to sleep.[6]

PREVENTIVE SERVICES—PRESCHOOLERS (AGES 1 TO 4 YEARS)

Example

A healthy 3-year-old girl is brought in by her parents for a wellness visit—health evaluation and preventive counseling. The clinician takes

TABLE 7.5	Clinical Preventive Services for Infants (<1 Year of Age)	
Screening	**Resources for Doctors**	**Resources for Patients**
Hearing	Hearing tests: American Academy of Pediatrics (http://www.medicalhomeinfo.org/Screening/hearing.html)	
Height, weight, and head circumference	Growth and head circumference charts (http://www.cdc.gov/growthcharts/clinical_charts.htm) *Note:* Overweight: 85th–95th percentile; obese: 95th+ percentile	Same charts may be printed out in color
Counseling		
Development	Growth charts; health care provider resource kit and milestone checklist (http://www.cdc.gov/ncbddd/actearly/hcp/index.html)	Interactive tool to check milestones (CDC; http://www.cdc.gov/ncbddd/actearly/milestones)
Nutrition	Breastfeeding interventions for health care providers (CDC; http://www.cdc.gov/breastfeeding/pdf/breastfeeding_interventions.pdf)	Breastfeeding information/assistance (U.S. Health and Human Services; http://www.womenshealth.gov/Breastfeeding)
Injury prevention/safety	Injury Fact Book (CDC; http://www.cdc.gov/Injury/Publications/FactBook/) Violence Prevention (including child abuse) (http://www.cdc.gov/ViolencePrevention/index.html)	Child safety checklist (see Chapter 10)

a complete history and performs a comprehensive physical examination with review of systems. He evaluates the child's growth and development, including height, weight, and developmental milestones. He discusses injury prevention, including correct use of the car seat, appropriate nutrition, and any risk factors identified, along with methods to reduce or eliminate them.

Table 7.6 summarizes the recommendations made by the USPSTF on appropriate screening and counseling for preschoolers. Growth, development, and vision should be screened to ensure preschoolers are in good health. Counseling on nutrition and injury prevention is particularly important for this age group. Lifelong dietary habits begin to be developed in toddlers. Unintentional injuries are the leading cause of death in this age group and, disturbingly, homicide is among the top five causes of death.[7,8] The American Academy of Pediatrics has developed a program, The Injury Prevention Program (TIPP), to assist physicians in advising parents and children on injury prevention.[9] Application of counseling on injury prevention for children to chiropractic practice has also been described in detail.[8] The CDC's Injury Fact Book is a useful resource for both clinicians and parents of children of all ages.[10]

PREVENTIVE SERVICES—MIDDLE CHILDHOOD (AGES 5 TO 11 YEARS)

Example

A healthy 11-year-old boy is brought in by his father for health supervision and

TABLE 7.6	Clinical Preventive Services for Preschoolers (Ages 1 to 4 Years)	
Screening	**Resources for Doctors**	**Resources for Patient**
Height, weight	Growth charts (http://www.cdc.gov/growthcharts/clinical_charts.htm) *Note:* Overweight: 85th–95th percentile; obese: 95th+ percentile	Same charts may be printed out in color
Vision	Age 3–4 y. Article on preschool vision screening for physicians (http://www.aafp.org/afp/980901ap/broderic.html)	Patient handout on strabismus (http://www.aafp.org/afp/980901ap/980901a.html)
Counseling		
Development	Growth charts; health care provider resource kit and milestone checklist (http://www.cdc.gov/ncbddd/actearly/hcp/index.html)	Interactive tool to check milestones (CDC; http://www.cdc.gov/ncbddd/actearly/milestones)
Nutrition	See Chapter 9 Nutrition resources for health care providers (CDC; http://www.cdc.gov/nutrition/professionals/index.html) *Fruit and Veggies—More Matters*: For health care providers (http://www.cdc.gov/nutrition/everyone/fruitsvegetables/index.html)	*"Nutrition for Everyone."* Basic nutrition information (CDC; http://www.cdc.gov/nutrition/everyone/index.html) Kid's Health—For Parents (http://kidshealth.org/parent/index.jsp?tracking=P_Home) *Fruit and Veggies—More Matters* (http://www.fruitsandveggiesmatter.gov)
Injury prevention/safety	Injury Fact Book (CDC; http://www.cdc.gov/Injury/Publications/FactBook) Violence Prevention (including child abuse) (http://www.cdc.gov/ViolencePrevention/index.html)	Child safety checklists (http://www.cpsc.gov/cpscpub/pubs/chld_sfy.html)

evaluation. The clinician takes a complete family, social, and medical history, including a review of systems. She performs a comprehensive physical examination, including height, weight, blood pressure, and dental health screening. She provides guidance to the child and his father about good health habits and self-care, including adequate physical activity, proper nutrition, and maintenance of healthy weight. Risk factors and methods to address them are discussed with the child and parent.

Table 7.7 summarizes the recommendations made by the USPSTF on appropriate screening and counseling for this age group. By middle childhood, it becomes particularly important to screen children for overweight and obesity (although these may emerge at even younger ages). Thus, counseling on physical activity should be added to counseling on nutrition and injury prevention for this age group, to develop a life-long habit of being physically active. Children in middle childhood should be included in the counseling sessions, along with their parents.

TABLE 7.7	Clinical Preventive Services for Middle Childhood (Ages 5 to 11)	
Screening	**Resources for Doctors**	**Information and Resources for Patients**
Height, weight	Growth charts (http://www.cdc.gov/growthcharts/clinical_charts.htm) *Note:* Overweight: 85th–95th percentile; obese: 95th+ percentile	Same charts may be printed out in color
Counseling		
Development	Developmental milestones and parenting advice (CDC; http://cdc.gov/ncbddd/child)	Developmental milestones and parenting advice (CDC; http://www.cdc.gov/ncbddd/child)
Physical activity	Guidelines on physical activity (http://www.cdc.gov/healthyyouth/physicalactivity/guidelines.htm) Weight management (http://www.nhlbi.nih.gov/health/public/heart/obesity/wecan)	Brochure on physical activity for families (http://www.cdc.gov/healthyyouth/physicalactivity/toolkit/factsheet_pa_guidelines_families.pdf)
Nutrition	See Chapter 9 Nutrition resources for health care providers (CDC; http://www.cdc.gov/nutrition/professionals/index.html) *Fruit and Veggies—More Matters*: For health care providers (http://www.cdc.gov/nutrition/everyone/fruitsvegetables/index.html)	"Nutrition for Everyone." Basic nutrition information (CDC; http://www.cdc.gov/nutrition/everyone/index.html) Kid's Health—For Parents (http://kidshealth.org/parent/index.jsp?tracking=P_Home) *Fruit and Veggies—More Matters* (http://www.cdc.gov/nutrition/everyone/fruitsvegetables/index.html)
Injury prevention/safety	Injury Fact Book (CDC; http://www.cdc.gov/Injury/Publications/FactBook) Violence Prevention (including child abuse; http://www.cdc.gov/ViolencePrevention/index.html)	Child safety checklists (http://www.cpsc.gov/cpscpub/pubs/chld_sfy.html)

PREVENTIVE SERVICES—TEENS (AGES 12 TO 17 YEARS)

Example

A healthy 16-year-old girl presents for health supervision and evaluation. A complete family, social, and medical history is taken along with a comprehensive physical examination, including height, weight, blood pressure, and dental health. A complete review of systems is performed. Growth, development, and behavior are assessed, including screening for major depressive disorder. Anticipatory guidance is provided regarding health habits and self-care, including physical activity and good diet. Risk factors are discussed, including driving responsibly, using seat belts, and safe sex.

(continued)

Table 7.8 summarizes the recommendations made by the USPSTF on appropriate screening and counseling. Added to the need for screening for development and appropriate body mass index (BMI) is the need to screen teens for depression, which appears to be increasing in prevalence. Teens should be the focus of counseling, either with or without their parents, depending upon the individual situation and local informed consent requirements. Teens need information on healthy diet, physical activity, and injury prevention—particularly in sports and in driving or cycling—and nonjudgmental, factual information on sexual behavior and substance use.

PREVENTIVE SERVICES—ADULTS (AGES 18 TO 39 YEARS)

Example

A healthy 33-year-old man presents for a complete health evaluation and physical examination. He has no specific complaints. The clinician takes a complete family, social, and medical history along with a comprehensive physical examination, including vital signs and BMI. He performs a complete review of systems, including screening for depression. If risk factors for heart disease are present, the clinician recommends cholesterol and blood glucose screening. Risk factors, including poor diet, tobacco use, and alcohol abuse, are identified, and interventions to reduce them are discussed.

Table 7.9 summarizes the recommendations made by the USPSTF on appropriate screening and counseling for adults. Screening should be done to detect abnormal BMI, blood pressure, cholesterol, and blood glucose, and for women, cervical cancer. Furthermore, patients should be screened through questionnaires or interviews about diet, tobacco use, alcohol abuse, and depression. Instruments for assessing these items are mentioned in this chapter.

PREVENTIVE SERVICES—MIDDLE-AGED ADULTS (AGES 40 TO 64 YEARS)

Example

A 49-year-old woman with no complaints presents for a complete health evaluation and physical examination. A complete family, social, and medical history is taken along with a comprehensive physical examination, including height, weight, BMI, and blood pressure. A complete review of systems is performed, including screening for depression. Cholesterol, diabetes, breast cancer, and cervical cancer screenings are recommended. Risk factors are identified, including poor diet, tobacco use, alcohol use, and injury prevention, including using seat belts. Counseling is provided for the risk factors identified.

Table 7.10 summarizes the recommendations made by the USPSTF on appropriate screening and counseling for middle-aged adults. Screening for this age group is similar to that for younger adults, with the addition of screening for colorectal cancer and, for women, breast cancer and osteoporosis, as detailed in Table 7.10. Counseling recommendations are basically the same for these age groups as well.

PREVENTIVE SERVICES—OLDER ADULTS (AGES 65 YEARS AND OLDER)

Example

A 70-year-old male with no complaint presents for a complete health evaluation and physical examination. A complete past, family, and social history is taken along with a comprehensive physical examination, including vital signs and BMI. A complete review of systems is performed, including screening for depression. Risk factors are identified, including weight loss, tobacco use, alcohol abuse, and risk of falls. Screening is indicated for abdominal aortic aneurysm, cholesterol, and colorectal cancer.

Table 7.11 summarizes the recommendations made by the USPSTF on appropriate screening and counseling for preschoolers. Screening for this age group is the same as for middle-aged adults, with the addition of screening for aortic aneurysms for men aged 65 to 75 years who have ever smoked. Counseling is also the same, with the addition of advice on fall prevention and prevention of elder abuse.

TABLE 7.8	Clinical Preventive Services for Teens (Ages 12 to 17 Years)	
Screening	**Resources for Doctors**	**Information and Resources for Patient**
Height, weight	Growth charts (http://www.cdc.gov/growthcharts/clinical_charts.htm) *Note:* Overweight: 85th–95th percentile; obese: 95th+ percentile	Same charts may be printed out in color
Depression	Only screen for depression if adequate resources are available locally for treatment PHQ-9 depression instrument and instructions (http://steppingup.washington.edu/keys/documents/phq-9.pdf) PHQ-p for adolescents (https://provider.ghc.org/open/caringForOurMembers/patientHealthEducation/depressQ.pdf)	
Counseling		
Development	Developmental milestones and parenting advice (CDC; http://cdc.gov/ncbddd/child)	Developmental milestones and parenting advice (CDC; http://www.cdc.gov/ncbddd/child)
Physical activity	Guidelines on physical activity (http://www.cdc.gov/healthyyouth/physicalactivity/guidelines.htm) Weight management (www.nhlbi.nih.gov/health/public/heart/obesity/wecan)	Brochure on physical activity for families (http://www.cdc.gov/healthyyouth/physicalactivity/toolkit/factsheet_pa_guidelines_families.pdf)
Nutrition	See Chapter 9 Nutrition resources for health care providers (CDC; http://www.cdc.gov/nutrition/professionals/index.html) *Fruit and Veggies—More Matters*: for health care providers (http://www.cdc.gov/nutrition/everyone/fruitsvegetables/index.html)	"Nutrition for Everyone" (CDC; http://www.cdc.gov/nutrition/everyone/index.html) Kid's Health—for Parents (http://kidshealth.org/parent/index.jsp?tracking=P_Home) *Fruit and Veggies—More Matters* (http://www.fruitsandveggiesmatter.gov)
Injury prevention/safety	Injury Fact Book (CDC; http://www.cdc.gov/Injury/Publications/FactBook) Injury prevention for teens (http://origin2.cdc.gov/ncbddd/child/adolescence.htm) Violence Prevention (including child abuse; http://www.cdc.gov/ViolencePrevention/index.html)	Child safety checklists (http://www.cpsc.gov/cpscpub/pubs/chld_sfy.html)
STDs/HIV	Questions on STDs (http://www.cdcnpin.org/scripts/std/index.asp.)	Teens/parents may use link (http://www.cdc.gov/std/phq.htm)

PHQ, patient health questionnaire.

TABLE 7.9	Clinical Preventive Services for Adults (Ages 18 to 39 Years)	
Screening	**Resources for Doctors**	**Information and Resources for Patients**
BMI	Overweight/obesity calculator, Figure 6.1 BMI Calculator (http://www.nhlbisupport.com/bmi/bmicalc.htm) BMI chart (http://www.nhlbi.nih.gov/guidelines/obesity/bmi_tbl.htm)	Patient may also use these links BMI Calculator (http://www.nhlbisupport.com/bmi/bmicalc.htm) BMI chart (http://www.nhlbi.nih.gov/guidelines/obesity/bmi_tbl.htm)
Blood pressure	—	Patient information on hypertension: (http://www.heart.org/HEARTORG/Conditions/HighBloodPressure/High-Blood-Pressure-or-Hypertension_UCM_002020_SubHomePage.jsp)
Cholesterol	Screening for all men 35+ y, otherwise screening only if risk factors for heart disease are present Overview of cholesterol evaluation and treatment from National Heart, Lung, and Blood Institute (http://www.nhlbi.nih.gov/guidelines/cholesterol/atp3xsum.pdf)	Patient education materials from National Library of Medicine (http://www.nlm.nih.gov/medlineplus/cholesterol.html)
Blood glucose	Obese patients and/or at risk for heart disease. American Diabetes Association defines diabetes as fasting plasma glucose level of ≥126 mg/dL, and recommends confirmation with a repeated screening test on a separate day	Patient information from National Institute of Diabetes and Digestive and Kidney Diseases (http://diabetes.niddk.nih.gov/dm/pubs/type1and2/what.htm)
Cervical cancer	Women over 35 y, every 3 y	Patient information—online booklet from National Cancer Institute (http://www.cancer.gov/cancertopics/wyntk/cervix)

Risk Factor Identification

Diet	Patients with high cholesterol or heart disease/diabetes risk: Screening, Figure 6.2	—
Tobacco	Screening (Table 6.2)	—
Alcohol	Screening (See Chapter 11; http://alcoholism.about.com/od/tests/a/screening.htm) Treatment referrals (http://www.samhsa.gov/data/dasis.htm)	Online quizzes and info (http://www.alcoholscreening.org and http://alcoholism.about.com/od/problem/a/blquiz1.htm)
Depression	Only screen for depression if adequate resources are available locally for treatment. PHQ-9 depression instrument and instructions (http://steppingup.washington.edu/keys/documents/phq-9.pdf)	—

TABLE 7.9	Clinical Preventive Services for Adults (Ages 18 to 39 Years) (*continued*)	
Screening	**Resources for Doctors**	**Information and Resources for Patients**
Counseling		
Physical activity	American College of Sports Medicine pre-exercise health assessment http://www.myexerciseplan.com/assessment/ Screening, Table 6.3	Recommendations and tips on physical activity (CDC; http://cdc.gov/ physicalactivity/everyone/guidelines/ index.html)
Nutrition	*Fruit and Veggies —More Matters*: for health care providers (http://www.cdc.gov/nutrition/ everyone/fruitsvegetables/index.html)	"Nutrition for Everyone." Basic nutrition information (CDC; http:// www.cdc.gov/nutrition/everyone/ index.html) *Fruit and Veggies—More Matters* (http:// www.fruitsandveggiesmatter.gov)
Tobacco	See Chapter 12	http://www.cdc.gov/tobacco/quit_ smoking/index.htm
Weight management	Overweight and obese patients; see Chapter 10	From USDHHS: Program on healthy weight management (http://www.cdc. gov/healthyweight/losing_weight/ index.html)
Injury prevention/ safety (including partner abuse)	Injury Fact Book (CDC; http://www.cdc.gov/ Injury/Publications/FactBook) Violence Prevention (including domestic violence; http://www.cdc.gov/ ViolencePrevention/index.html) Screening for domestic violence (http://www. ncjrs.gov/pdffiles1/nij/188564.pdf) Guidelines for health care providers on screening for and responding to domestic violence (http://www.endabuse.org/userfiles/ file/Consensus.pdf)	—

TABLE 7.10	Clinical Preventive Services for Middle-Aged Adults (Ages 40 to 64 Years)	
Screening	**Resources for Doctors**	**Information and Resources for Patients**
BMI	Overweight/obesity calculator, Figure 7.1. BMI calculator (http://www.nhlbisupport.com/bmi/bmicalc.htm) BMI chart (http://www.nhlbi.nih.gov/guidelines/obesity/bmi_tbl.htm)	Patient may also use these links: BMI calculator (http://www.nhlbisupport.com/bmi/bmicalc.htm) BMI chart (http://www.nhlbi.nih.gov/guidelines/obesity/bmi_tbl.htm)
Blood pressure	—	Patient information on hypertension: http://www.heart.org/HEARTORG/Conditions/HighBloodPressure/High-Blood-Pressure-or-Hypertension_UCM_002020_SubHomePage.jsp
Cholesterol	Screening for all men and for women at risk up to age 45 y and all women over 45 y. Overview of cholesterol evaluation and treatment from National Heart, Lung, and Blood Institute (http://www.nhlbi.nih.gov/guidelines/cholesterol/atp3xsum.pdf)	Patient education materials from National Library of Medicine (http://www.nlm.nih.gov/medlineplus/cholesterol.html)
Blood glucose	Obese patients and/or at risk for heart disease. American Diabetes Association defines diabetes as fasting plasma glucose level of $\geq$126 mg/dL, and recommends confirmation with a repeated screening test on a separate day.	Patient information from National Institute of Diabetes and Digestive and Kidney Diseases (http://diabetes.niddk.nih.gov/dm/pubs/type1and2/what.htm)
Colorectal cancer	Age 50+: details at USPSTF (http://www.ahrq.gov/clinic/uspstf08/colocancer/colors.htm)	
Breast cancer	Mammography for women every 2 y starting at age 50 y	
Cervical cancer	PAP test for women every 3 y	Patient information—online booklet from National Cancer Institute (http://www.cancer.gov/cancertopics/wyntk/cervix)
Osteoporosis	Women aged 60+ at risk every 2 y or more; calculate risk with World Health Organization screening questionnaire (http://www.shef.ac.uk/FRAX/tool.jsp?locationValue=9)	

TABLE 7.10	Clinical Preventive Services for Middle-Aged Adults (Ages 40 to 64 Years) (*continued*)	
Screening	**Resources for Doctors**	**Information and Resources for Patients**
Risk Factor Identification		
Diet	Patients with high cholesterol or heart disease/diabetes risk: see Figure 6.2 for screening.	
Tobacco	See Table 7.4 for screening	
Alcohol	See Chapter 12 for screening; for referrals for treatment, see http://www.samhsa.gov/data/dasis.htm	
Depression	Only screen for depression if adequate resources are available locally for treatment. PHQ-9 depression instrument and instructions (http://steppingup.washington.edu/keys/documents/phq-9.pdf)	
Counseling		
Physical activity	American College of Sports Medicine pre-exercise health assessment (http://www.myexerciseplan.com/assessment) See Table 7.3 for screening	Recommendations and tips on physical activity (CDC; http://cdc.gov/physicalactivity/everyone/guidelines/index.html and http://www.easyforyou.info/index.asp)
Nutrition	*Fruit and Veggies* —More Matters: for health care providers (http://www.cdc.gov/nutrition/everyone/fruitsvegetables/index.html) See Figure 6.2 for screening	*Nutrition for Everyone.*" Basic nutrition information (CDC; http://www.cdc.gov/nutrition/everyone/index.html) *Fruit and Veggies—More Matters* (http://www.fruitsandveggiesmatter.gov)
Tobacco	See Chapter 12	http://www.cdc.gov/tobacco/quit_smoking/index.htm
Weight management	Overweight and obese patients; see Chapter 10	From USDHHS: Program on healthy weight management (http://www.cdc.gov/healthyweight/losing_weight/index.html)
Injury prevention/safety (including partner and elder abuse)	Injury Fact Book (CDC; http://www.cdc.gov/Injury/Publications/FactBook/) Violence Prevention (including domestic violence and elder abuse; http://www.cdc.gov/ViolencePrevention/index.html) Screening for domestic violence (http://www.ncjrs.gov/pdffiles1/nij/188564.pdf) Guidelines for health care providers on screening for and responding to domestic violence (http://www.endabuse.org/userfiles/file/Consensus.pdf)	

TABLE 7.11	Clinical Preventive Services for Older Adults (Ages 65 and Older)	
Screening	**Resources for Doctors**	**Information and Resources for Patients**
BMI	Overweight/obesity calculator, Figure 6.1 BMI Calculator (http://www.nhlbisupport.com/bmi/bmicalc.htm) BMI chart (http://www.nhlbi.nih.gov/guidelines/obesity/bmi_tbl.htm)	Patient may also use these links
Blood pressure	—	Patient information on hypertension: http://www.heart.org/HEARTORG/Conditions/HighBloodPressure/High-Blood-Pressure-or-Hypertension_UCM_002020_SubHomePage.jsp
Cholesterol	Screening for all men and for women at risk. Overview of cholesterol evaluation and treatment from National Heart, Lung and Blood Institute (http://www.nhlbi.nih.gov/guidelines/cholesterol/atp3xsum.pdf)	Patient education materials from National Library of Medicine (http://www.nlm.nih.gov/medlineplus/cholesterol.html)
Blood glucose	Obese patients and/or at risk for heart disease American Diabetes Association defines diabetes as fasting plasma glucose level $\geq$126 mg/dL and recommends confirmation with a repeated screening test on a separate day.	Patient information from National Institute of Diabetes, Digestive and Kidney Disease (http://diabetes.niddk.nih.gov/dm/pubs/type1and2/what.htm)
Breast cancer	Mammography for women every 2 y up to age 75	
Colorectal cancer	Ages 50–75; details at USPSTF (http://www.ahrq.gov/clinic/uspstf08/colocancer/colors.htm)	
Aortic aneurysm	Men 65–75 who have ever smoked; details at USPSTF (http://www.ahrq.gov/clinic/uspstf05/aaascr/aaars.htm)	
Osteoporosis	Women very 2 y or more; calculate risk with World Health Organization screening questionnaire (http://www.shef.ac.uk/FRAX/tool.jsp?locationValue=9)	
Risk Factor Identification		
Diet	Patients with high cholesterol or heart disease/diabetes risks Information on dietary fat: (http://cdc.gov/nutrition/everyone/basics/fat/index.html)	
Tobacco	See Table 7.2 for screening	
Alcohol	For referrals for treatment (http://dasis3.samhsa.gov)	
Depression	Only screen for depression if adequate resources are available locally for treatment. PHQ-9 depression instrument and instructions (http://steppingup.washington.edu/keys/documents/phq-9.pdf)	

TABLE 7.11	Clinical Preventive Services for Older Adults (Ages 65 and Older) *(continued)*	
Screening	**Resources for Doctors**	**Information and Resources for Patients**
Counseling		
Physical activity	American College of Sports Medicine pre-exercise health assessment (http://www.myexerciseplan.com/assessment) See Table 6.3 for screening	Recommendations and tips on physical activity (CDC; http://cdc.gov/physicalactivity/everyone/guidelines/index.html and http://www.easyforyou.info/index.asp)
Nutrition	*Fruit and Veggies—More Matters*: for health care providers (http://www.fruitsandveggiesmatter.gov/health_professionals/educational_materials.html) See Figure 6.2 for screening	"Nutrition for Everyone." Basic nutrition information (CDC; http://www.cdc.gov/nutrition/everyone/index.html) *Fruit and Veggies—More Matters* (http://www.fruitsandveggiesmatter.gov)
Tobacco	See Chapter 12	http://www.cdc.gov/tobacco/quit_smoking/index.htm
Weight management	Overweight and obese patients; see Chapter 10	From USDHHS: program on healthy weight management (http://www.cdc.gov/healthyweight/losing_weight/index.html)
Fall prevention	CDC information on falls (http://www.cdc.gov/HomeandRecreationalSafety/Falls/adultfalls.html)	Brochures for patients (http://www.cdc.gov/HomeandRecreationalSafety/Falls/fallsmaterial.html)
Injury prevention including partner and elder abuse)	Injury Fact Book (CDC; http://www.cdc.gov/Injury/Publications/FactBook) Violence Prevention (including domestic violence and elder abuse; http://www.cdc.gov/ViolencePrevention/index.html) Screening for domestic violence (http://www.ncjrs.gov/pdffiles1/nij/188564.pdf) Guidelines for health care providers on screening for and responding to domestic violence (http://www.endabuse.org/userfiles/file/Consensus.pdf)	—

Literature Cited

1. USPSTF. *Guide to Clinical Preventive Services.* Washington, DC: Agency for Healthcare Research and Quality; 2009.
2. American Medical Association. *CPT 2010 Professional Edition.* American Medical Association; 2010.
3. Nicoletti B. Reimbursement for clinical preventive services. In: Woolf S, Jonas S, Kaplan-Liss E, ed. *Health Promotion and Disease Prevention in Clinical Practice.* 2nd ed. Philadelphia, PA: Wolters Kluwer; 2008:563–581.
4. Hawk CSM, Schneider M, Ferrance RJ, et al. Best practices recommendations for chiropractic care for infants, children, and adolescents: results of a consensus process. *J Manipulative Physiol Ther.* 2009;32(8):639–647 .
5. Khorsan R, Smith M, Hawk C, et al. A public health Immunization Resource Website for chiropractors: discussion of current issues and future challenges for evidence-based initiatives for the chiropractic profession. *J Manipulative Physiol Ther.* 2009;32(6):500–504.
6. Colson ER, Rybin D, Smith LA, et al. Trends and factors associated with infant sleeping position: the National Infant Sleep Position Study, 1993-2007. *Arch Pediatr Adolesc Med.* 2009;163(12):1122–1128.
7. Borse N, Gilchrist J, Dellinger AM, et al. CDC *Childhood Injury Report: Patterns of Unintentional Injuries among 0–19 Year Olds in the United States, 2000–2006.* Atlanta, GA: Centers for Disease Control and Prevention; 2008.
8. Hawk C. Counseling on unintentional injury prevention: how chiropractors can help keep children safe. J Clin Chiropractic Pediatr. 2009;10(2):671–675.
9. Gardner HG. Office-based counseling for unintentional injury prevention. *Pediatrics.* 2007;119(1):202–206.
10. National Center for Injury Prevention and Control. *CDC Injury Fact Book.* Atlanta, GA: Centers for Disease Control and Prevention; 2006.

CHAPTER 8

Counseling and Coaching on Physical Activity

Ronald D. Williams, Jr.

Maintaining a physically active lifestyle is undoubtedly one of the most important preventive measures a person can take. Physical activity has been linked to multiple healthy outcomes such as weight control, reduced risk for cardiovascular disease and diabetes, improved mental health, fall prevention, among many other benefits.[1–4] These are only a few of the many health protections afforded to the physically active; therefore, health care practitioners have a responsibility to prescribe and encourage physical activity to all patients, with particular interest for those in need. With an aging population and growing health care costs, it is vital to our communities that health care providers promote preventive behaviors among patients. It is quite possible that physical activity may be the most important behavior in chronic disease control and prevention. While some health care providers do discuss exercise and activity with patients, research indicates that patients need more advice than what is currently offered.[5,6] The goal of the health care practitioner should be to "inspire action" from the patient; therefore, simply telling a patient to exercise or even providing basic education may not be enough.[7] Luckily, research in the areas of behavior change, health communication, and patient–practitioner relationship has highlighted promising techniques that may assist in getting the patients moving. This chapter will:

- Highlight the importance of physical activity as a preventive behavior.
- Examine the basic physical activity guidelines as proposed by major U.S. health organizations.
- Explore two behavior change models used in health promotion that may assist health care providers in better assessing a patient's influences and readiness for physical activity.
- Discuss counseling and advocacy strategies that the health care provider may implement to increase physical activity participation among patients.

BASIC PHYSICAL ACTIVITY GUIDELINES

It's nearly universally known that exercise is good medicine, yet many people simply are not as physically active as they should be. Although not the primary responsibility, many health care providers find themselves in the role of exercise counselor as they attempt to encourage patients to increase physical activity, often to alleviate symptoms or prevent further illness or infirmity. To assist health care providers, this section will share the basic guidelines for physical activity as declared by leading health organizations in the US.

Defining exercise standards can be difficult due to the physiological differences among age groups and varying health conditions that affect the population, but there exists an extensive body of research on physical activity benchmarks. In an effort to synthesize the research related to physical activity, the U.S. Department of Health and Human Services (DHHS) published the *2008 Physical Activity Guidelines for Americans* to be used as a tool for both health professionals and policymakers.[8] This document provides the health care professional with information about physical activity across the life span, including details on injury prevention and safety strategies. Although most people, both providers and patients alike, know that physical activity is a healthful behavior, the guidelines focus on the major research findings in an attempt to translate research into practice. The following represents a summary of key recommendations from the guidelines.

General Guidelines

A distinction is made in the guidelines to assist in clarifying an often misunderstood concept related to physical activity—activities of daily life versus organized, sustained exercise bouts. The DHHS guidelines refer to activities of daily life as baseline activity, such as standing, slow walking, or lifting light objects.[8] Baseline activity differs from sustained activity in that it is often low

TABLE 8.1	Classification of Total Weekly Amounts of Aerobic Physical Activity		
Levels of Physical Activity	**Range of Moderate-Intensity Minutes a Week**	**Summary of Overall Health Benefits**	**Comments**
Inactive	No activity beyond baseline	None	Being inactive is unhealthy
Low	Activity beyond baseline but fewer than 150 min/wk	Some	Low levels of activity are clearly preferable to an inactive lifestyle
Medium	150 min to 300 min/wk	Substantial	Activity at the high end of this range has additional and more extensive health benefits than activity at the low end
High	More than 300 min/wk	Additional	Current science does not allow researchers to identify an upper limit of activity above which there are no additional health benefits

Source: From U.S. of Health and Human Services. 2008 Physical Activity Guidelines for Americans. http://www.health.gov/paguidelines. Accessed February 29, 2011, with permission.

in intensity and duration. Extended activities are referred to as health-enhancing physical activities, with examples being brisk walking, yoga, weight lifting, or dancing.[8] These activities differ in the physiological impact on the body; therefore, the health benefits derived are quite different. The DHHS document provides guidelines on health-enhancing activities, but does encourage the promotion of additional baseline activities among the population because such activities may improve bone health, burn more calories, and create a more supportive culture for physical activity.[8] The baseline versus health-enhancing issue should be important to health care providers delivering physical activity education as patients may not understand the difference. Many people cannot accurately assess their personal participation in physical activity,[9–11] so patients may consider baseline activities to be sufficient for health improvements. Although health care providers should encourage increased baseline activities, it is important to educate patients on the need for health-enhancing exercise. It may be of use to health care providers to use the DHHS table below to quickly assess the current physical activity level of patients (Table 8.1).

Health-Enhancing Activity for All Ages

Owing to physiological differences, activity needs vary as people age. The DHHS guidelines provide suggestions for age groups from children to older adults, including considerations for pregnancy or disability. Though the intensity, frequency, duration, and type of activity may change throughout the life span, one common guideline is that people should avoid inactivity; the guidelines specifically state, "Some physical activity is better than none."[8] Sedentary behaviors, regardless of age, increase the likelihood of chronic disease and illness; therefore, a healthy, active lifestyle is necessary from childhood to older adulthood. In addition, physical activity for all ages should include both aerobic and strength-training activities to maximize health benefits. Table 8.2 provides key guidelines for all ages.[8]

NOTE ON PHYSICAL ACTIVITY AMONG YOUTH

Despite the documented health benefits, many children and adolescents are not physically active.[12] Furthermore, youth (especially females) tend to show a reduction in physically active behaviors as they enter adolescence.[13,14] Although research is limited, it may be a safe assumption that participation in regular physical activity during childhood increases the likelihood of becoming an active adult. What is known is that inactive children have an increased likelihood of becoming inactive adults, leading to increased risk of chronic health concerns.[15] To maximize the lifelong benefits of being physically active, health care providers should be prepared to educate both youth patients and their parents on the rewards of being physically active.

TABLE 8.2	U.S. DHHS Key Guidelines for Physical Activity of Americans (All Ages)

Adults (18 to 64 Years)

Some physical activity is better than none; therefore, adults should avoid inactivity

Most health benefits occur with at least 150 min/week of moderate-intensity physical activity, or 75 min/week of high-intensity physical activity

Health benefits increase as activity levels increase. More extensive health benefits occur with at least 300 min/week of moderate-intensity physical activity, or 150 min/week of high-intensity physical activity

Additional health benefits are gained from performing moderate- or high-intensity muscle-strengthening activities involving all major muscle groups on 2 or more days per week. The American College of Sports Medicine and the American Heart Association recommend the healthy adult participate twice a week in 8 to 10 strength-training exercises while performing 8 to 12 repetitions of each[a]

Older Adults (65 Years and Above)

Guidelines for older adults are the same as those for adults with the following additions:

If older adults cannot perform 150 min/week of moderate-intensity physical activity, they should be physically active as their abilities allow

Older adults should perform activities that improve balance to reduce fall risk

Level of effort for exercise should be determined based on the older adult's level of fitness

Consideration of chronic conditions should be taken into account to understand how those conditions may affect physical activity of the older adult

Children and Adolescents (6 to 17 Years)

Children should participate in 60 min of daily physical activity

Most of the 60 min of daily physical activity should be moderate- or high-intensity aerobic activity, with at least 3 days/week of high-intensity activity

As part of the 60 min, children and adolescents should perform muscle-strengthening activity at least 3 days/week

As part of the 60 min, children and adolescents should perform bone-strengthening activity at least 3 days/week

Children and adolescents should be offered a variety of age-appropriate activity options to make the experience enjoyable

[a]Data taken from Ref. 4.

Source: From U.S. of Health and Human Services. 2008 Physical Activity Guidelines for Americans. http://www.health.gov/paguidelines. Accessed February 29, 2011, with permission.

As shown in Table 8.2, the DHHS guidelines suggest three types of activities for children: Aerobic, muscle-strengthening, and bone-strengthening. Participation in these activities at an early age may prevent health problems later in life.[8]

HEALTH BEHAVIOR THEORY AND BARRIERS TO PHYSICAL ACTIVITY

Most of the general public would agree that basic health behaviors are good for us: Eating right, exercising, and avoiding tobacco. However, as anyone who has attempted to make a behavior change can attest, knowing that a behavior can be beneficial to our health and actually performing that behavior consistently are quite different. The process of changing a behavior is complex, primarily because of the multifarious nature of behavior itself. The root of behavioral choices lies in the influences that impact a person's decision to perform or avoid such actions. Behavioral research has highlighted the varying influences on health choices that facilitate or impede behavioral change, yet people rarely attempt to address the influences when attempting to change a behavior.

Similarly, when health care providers advise patients to increase physical activity, how frequently are the behavioral influences discussed? Are attempts made to alter the influences or simply alter the behavior? For example, a health care provider may recommend to a slightly overweight patient that he or she walk for 30 minutes each day. The provider may even discuss the benefits of this activity and how it can help other health conditions. What the provider may not address are the factors that enhance or prohibit the patient from daily walking. Such factors may be financial status, family dynamics, time management, or any other barrier perceived by the patient. Perhaps the patient lives in a neighborhood that is not pedestrian-friendly (no sidewalks, no city parks, high crime) and simply cannot afford the monthly gym membership fee. Perhaps the patient does not perceive that an exercise regimen will fit into the time constraints on daily life. In fact, lack of time is the most frequently reported barrier to physical activity participation.[16-20] The question becomes: How can health care providers address behavioral influences to assist patients in making healthy behavior changes?

One tool that health care providers can borrow from the field of health promotion is the use of behavioral theory. Theory exists to explain behavior and serves to help individuals make healthy changes.[21] Explanatory theory describes behavioral influences such as attitudes, values, social norms, and so on. Other theories assist health educators in the development of appropriate health promotion programs. While many of these theories are useful in community health programs, they can be valuable tools for the health care provider when addressing individual patients. Regarding the promotion of physical activity, it may be beneficial to the health care provider to examine a patient's behavior from two theoretical perspectives: Social ecological model and stages of change.

Social Ecological Model

Early research on the ecology of behavior suggested that life is operationalized through a system of reciprocal causation between a person and the containing environment.[22,23] Exploring ecology in health promotion, it was suggested that behavior is affected by influences at both the micro and macro levels.[24-28] The choice to participate in regular physical activity is a multifaceted behavior in which influence is drawn from various sources; therefore, an ecological approach of examining this behavior may be beneficial to providers and patients. The key concept in social ecology is that behavior is multifaceted, with social and environmental issues being impinging factors. The social ecological perspective of health suggests that behavior has five levels of influence: Intrapersonal, interpersonal, institutional/organizational, community, and public policy (Table 8.3). Each domain provides unique influences on behavior, in addition to creating a reciprocal cycle between the other domains and behavioral choices.

Substance abuse, nutrition, and physical activity are examples of health behaviors that have been explored through the social ecological perspective.[29-34] This framework allows the health educator to better understand the influences on complex behavior, thereby increasing the possibility of implementing successful health promotion programs and strategies. From the health care provider's standpoint, examining a patient's behavior from the ecological perspective allows for more in-depth communication, counseling, and barrier elimination. To maximize the impact of patient health education, providers must address behavioral influences. In addition, health care providers can play a large role in shaping the ecological influences of social norms and public policy through advocacy efforts.

Stages of Change Model

Research has indicated that practitioners do deliver health education to patients regarding physical activity[35-38]; yet, how frequently is readiness to change behavior evaluated? If a patient is simply not ready to begin an exercise program or has no intention of becoming more physically active, what is the purpose of spending time discussing exercise options with him or her? It may be of benefit to a practitioner to determine a patient's level of readiness to behavior change. This can be accomplished by examining behavior through the stages of change model.

While many health care providers focus on responding to acute health problems among patients, one of the roles of providers is to assist patients in making healthy behavior changes.[39,40] Examining a patient's behavior through stages allows the health care provider to better assist with the behavior change action plan. The basis of the stages of change model (officially titled Transtheoretical Model) is that behavior change is a time-consuming process rather than a single event.[21,38,41,42] At any given time, an individual may be in one of five different stages of readiness to change: Precontemplation, contemplation,

TABLE 8.3	Social Ecological Factors that Influence Physical Activity	
Social Ecological Level	**Type of Influence**	**Examples of Influence on PA Behaviors**
Intrapersonal factors	Characteristics include personal knowledge, attitudes, and beliefs concerning particular behaviors; issues of personal skill and self-concept	Belief that PA is healthy and needed for optimal wellness Self-efficacy in PA performance and skills Positive attitude toward PA participation
Interpersonal factors	Social networks including family, friends, and work groups	Family/friends support of PA behaviors Family participation in PA as a group
Organizational factors	Social practices with organizational characteristics, including the formal and informal rules and regulations for operation within the particular institution; organizational norms and changes of those norms can affect behavior of those individuals involved	Employer who supports PA initiatives as part of job (worksite wellness) Participation in organizations that support PA participation and initiatives (AHA or ACS PA events)
Community factors	Relationships among organizations, institutions, and informal networks within defined boundaries; includes the social standards or norms that exist within the community.	Residing in a community with access to PA options such as parks, sidewalks, bike lanes, etc. Community norms that accept PA among population (support of increased cycle traffic and pedestrians)
Policy factors	Policies and laws that are designed to protect the health of a community; policies for health protection include regulations for healthy actions, disease prevention, and disease control	Communities and/or states that enact laws/ordinances supporting PAs (bike lane ordinances; sidewalk ordinances) School policies that require daily PE for K-12 students

AHA, american heart association; ACS, american cancer society; PA, physical activity; PE, physical education.

Source: From Glanz, K, Rimer, B. *Theory at a glance: a guide for health promotion practice*. Bethesda, MD: National Cancer Institute; 1995, with permission; From McLeroy K, Bibeau D, Steckler A, et al. An ecological perspective on health promotion programs. *Health Educ Quar.* 1988;15:351–377, with permission.

preparation, action, and maintenance. Table 8.4 provides a brief description of each stage and gives examples of how a person at each stage may view physical activity participation. As most health care providers can attest, telling a patient to increase physical activity does not always mean he or she will do it. Part of the problem could be that providers are educating in one stage, while the patient actually resides in a different stage. For example, providing a detailed exercise prescription may work well for someone in the preparation phase, but it may provide little incentive to move someone from precontemplation into contemplation. Perhaps a better strategy to advance

the patient to the contemplation stage is a brief discussion about the patients' thoughts regarding exercise or a conversation about barriers to physical activity participation. This will certainly have more of an impact in stage progression than will providing information which the patient is not yet ready to think about.

Another important concept to remember regarding stages of change is that the stages are cyclical rather than linear.[21] Patients can progress through the stages while pursuing behavior change; however, they often enter and exit stages multiple times and frequently recycle through them again. When behavior change is discussed

TABLE 8.4	Stages of Change Model and How It Relates to Physical Activity	
Stages of Change	**Stage Definition**[a]	**Examples of Stage-Based Thoughts on Physical Activity (PA)**
Precontemplation	Unaware of problem; hasn't thought about change	Patient is not aware of personal health issues related to lack of PA Patient has no thoughts on how to incorporate more PA into lifestyle
Contemplation	Thinking about change in the near future	Patient is aware of need for increased PA Patient begins to consider PA participation in the next few months
Preparation	Making a plan to change a behavior	Patient becomes active in planning how to increase PA After exploring options, PA plans are created
Action	Implementation of specific action plans	Patient begins PA plan and is now participating in the behavior change
Maintenance	Continuation of desirable actions or repeating periodic recommended steps	Patient has remained physically active for at least 6 months PA is now a part of patient's regular lifestyle

[a]Data taken from Ref. 13.

with a patient, particularly related to physical activity, health care providers should attempt to assess readiness. As with social ecology, practical application of the stages of change will be discussed below.

Behavioral theories such as social ecology and stages of change are not definitive guides to explain behavior, but they are useful as maps to facilitate healthy change. Although more commonly applied in the public or community health promotion fields, there is certainly application within health care, particularly when assisting patients in changing physical activity behaviors. Considering the unique influences on exercise behavior and the variation in readiness of each patient, practitioners should seek to apply these theories in an effort to improve behavioral education. Behavior is multifaceted, so changing behavior frequently takes more than simple education.

Counseling Through Motivational Interviewing

As with any behavior change, an individual must possess some level of internal motivation to help sustain the change. For all the benefits of being physically active, motivating patients to build

more exercise into their lifestyle is difficult and frequently results in frustration by both patient and health care provider.[39] The disciplines of health promotion, clinical psychology, and even fitness training provide promising strategies to assist the health care provider in dealing with patient behavior change. One such strategy that has grown in use is motivational interviewing.[43] This patient-focused technique began in the 1980s as a practice in the treatment of alcohol problems,[44] but has shown promise in addressing a myriad of health-related issues from tobacco cessation to diabetes management.[45–48] Although motivational interviewing (MI) is primarily used in substance abuse and mental health counseling, there is great promise for this technique to help patients become more physically active.

The goal of MI is to facilitate behavior change in patients by helping them increase their motivation for change.[43,49] This approach is patient-centered; therefore, the provider must allow the patient to share his or her thoughts or feelings about the desired behavior change. It is common for patients to be ambivalent toward increasing physical activity, so MI strategies allow the patient to confront and express feelings about becoming more physically active.[50] Rather than being told to exercise more by an authority figure (the health care provider), the patient, through MI, has the opportunity to address barriers or fears and personally decide to make a behavior change. Key concepts in MI are collaboration between patient and provider, evocation of patient's thoughts, and autonomy of patient's behavioral choices.[51] The root of MI is to invoke the internal desire for behavior change in the patient. Although research is limited on the effect of MI among healthy patients, studies do indicate that this technique can improve physical activity among patients with various diagnosed conditions.[50,52–56]

Clinicians have reported that MI strategies are more effective than basic instructional approaches to behavior change, in addition to producing more satisfaction for both the patient and the health care provider.[57] The challenge in using MI in primary care is that it can be time-consuming and requires a specific skill set, which takes practice to master;[43] however, the potential benefits may be well worth the effort. Health care providers should seek to develop basic MI skills for implementing brief counseling on behavior change. Those skills include acknowledgment of inconsistency between the patient's behavior and values, practice of reflective listening, generating dialog using open-ended questions, displaying support of positive actions, and rolling with resistance.[43,57]

There are often intrinsic differences in how an individual behaves and how he or she may value that behavior. For example, a patient may not meet minimum guidelines for physical activity, but that does not mean that they do not value their health or the related physiological issues (obesity, overweight, hypertension, etc.). It could be highly possible that the patient's values have been displaced owing to the varying ecological influences in his or her life. Health care providers routinely see patients who express the desire to lose weight or be more physically active, yet have trouble putting this desire into practice. It is important for the practitioner to help the patients clarify the distinction between what they really want or value and how their current behaviors are affecting their health. Discussion and acknowledgment of the ecological influences can help patients discover these barriers and move them closer to values clarification and behavior change.

One simple tool that can assist the health care provider in beginning this values discussion with a patient is the agenda-setting chart.[39,58] The agenda-setting chart allows the patient to become actively involved with behavioral

decision making, thereby improving motivation for change through empowerment and self-efficacy.[59] Practitioners can use an agenda-setting chart to initiate discussion about physical activity and facilitate the patient in acknowledging barriers. Agenda-setting allows for open discussion of various behaviors affecting the patient's condition, but also encourages active participation from the patient in deciding which behavior changes will be attempted. It is important to note that patients and practitioners may not always agree on the most pressing behavioral issues, but it is essential to allow the patient to make decisions on behavior rather than have the practitioner give directives. Allowing a patient to make healthy changes in one area can increase self-efficacy and may lead him or her to adopt changes in behavior. For instance, if a patient is willing to make dietary changes, but resists increases in physical activity, practitioners should roll with this resistance while utilizing positive health communication techniques to encourage such dietary changes. As the patient progresses with healthy nutritional changes and as self-efficacy improves, the practitioner should continue to initiate dialogue about the other behaviors on the agenda. A sample agenda-setting chart and discussion script are included in Figure 8.1.

To continue dialogue and improve patient–provider communication, the health care provider should practice reflective listening and open-ended questioning during this discussion. Reflective listening is a communication strategy that allows the practitioner to fully understand the patient's thoughts and feelings without judgment, opinion, or offering advice.[60] The concept is central to the core of MI in that the behavioral change should be patient driven. When working through the behaviors on an agenda-setting chart, the provider must be cautious not to offer value-judgment statements about behavior into the discussion. The patient should be allowed to freely state his or her thoughts on their condition. The practitioner, however, should ask open-ended questions to determine social ecological influences on behavior. If changes can be made to these influences, the chance of a successful behavior change is improved.

If a patient is initially resistant to becoming more physically active, rather than continuously instructing them to exercise, a practitioner should accept that resistance, but continue using MI techniques to facilitate behavior change. Behavior is multifaceted, so behavior change is complex.

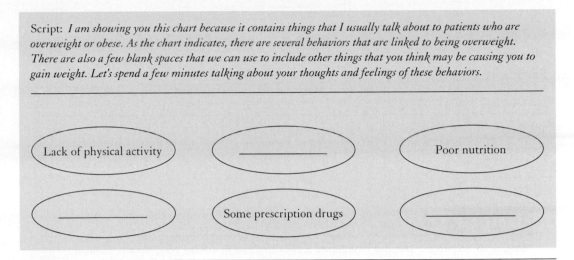

Script: I am showing you this chart because it contains things that I usually talk about to patients who are overweight or obese. As the chart indicates, there are several behaviors that are linked to being overweight. There are also a few blank spaces that we can use to include other things that you think may be causing you to gain weight. Let's spend a few minutes talking about your thoughts and feelings of these behaviors.

Lack of physical activity

_____

Poor nutrition

_____

Some prescription drugs

_____

Figure 8.1. A sample script and agenda-setting chart for patient discussion.

Providers should display positive support of a patient's healthy changes, another concept of MI. Every positive behavioral change increases self-efficacy, thereby potentially increasing the likelihood of additional healthy changes. With a patient-focused approach like MI, the patient drives the behavior change, yet the health care provider plays a vital role in facilitating that change by providing motivation in the course of positive interactions.

Readiness has been correlated with success in increasing physical activity.[61–63] It is quite possible that a patient just isn't ready to become more physically active despite the counseling and agenda-setting sessions. For clinical purposes, a health care provider may want to assess readiness to change, so how can this be accomplished? Another simple tool of MI is the readiness-to-change ruler, or simply, readiness ruler.[39,64,65] This tool allows the practitioner to easily determine how likely a patient is to currently begin a behavior change plan. A sample readiness ruler to measure physical activity readiness can be found in Figure 8.2. Quantifying readiness indicates the patient's stage of change to the practitioner, which then allows for more stage-appropriate communication. The practitioner's goal should be to assist the patient in moving toward the action stage; therefore, open-ended dialogue about physical activity should feature stage-specific questions from the practitioner. Examples of such questions are included in Table 8.5.

Building motivation among patients and facilitating the change toward a more active lifestyle should be a core goal for health care providers. As the DHHS physical activity guidelines suggest, the benefits of increasing activity levels far outweigh the potential risks.[8] The MI framework can be successfully applied by primary care professionals in clinical practice to build patients' motivation for physical activity by helping them to realize the value of an active lifestyle, develop appropriate health goals, and progress through the stages of change toward a more active, healthful lifestyle.

GOAL SETTING

While MI strategies should give health care providers the tools to help patients progress toward becoming more physically active, it is also important to remember that patients do not always know how to begin this type of behavior change. Although primary care providers may educate on physical activity,[5,6] very few assist patients with follow-through of exercise plans.[66,67] A key to establishing physical activity as a health behavior of importance to the health care provider is to assist in the development of appropriate goals. According to the goal-setting theory, the setting of specific goals indicates that a person has placed some value on the future outcome and therefore is more likely to continue progress toward that outcome.[68,69] The setting of a goal inherently creates more internal motivation for a person to achieve the outcome as opposed to setting a general guideline. In other words, if a patient sets a specific goal

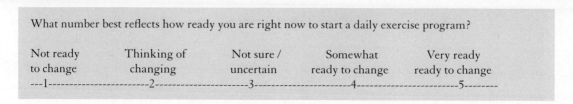

What number best reflects how ready you are right now to start a daily exercise program?

Not ready to change	Thinking of changing	Not sure / uncertain	Somewhat ready to change	Very ready ready to change
---1----------------------	---------2----------------------	----------3----------------------	------------4-------------------------	----------5--------

Figure 8.2. Sample Readiness-to-Change Ruler for physical activity. (From Leach R, Evans W, Williams R, et al. Grand rounds: teen with back pain complicated by obesity. J Clin Chiropr Pediatr. 2009;10(2):687–691, with permission.)

TABLE 8.5	Stage-Specific Questions Related to Physical Activity
Stages of Change	**Sample Questions a Health Care Provider May Ask a Patient**
Precontemplation	Have you tried to become more physically active in the past? What would have to happen to motivate you to increase your physical activity?
Contemplation	What are the challenges or barriers that keep you from becoming more physically active? What do you need to help you begin an exercise plan today? What is making you think about becoming more physically active at this time?
Preparation	What are your specific exercise plans? How are you addressing the barriers that we previously discussed?
Action	How is your physical activity plan progressing? What do you feel about your health now that you are more physically active?

Source: From Zimmerman GL, Olsen CG, Bosworth ME. A 'stages of change' approach to helping patients change behavior. *Am Fam Physician*. 2000;61:1409–1416, with permission.

to walk for 30 minutes each weekday for the next month, he or she is much more likely to accomplish this act than if he or she simply decided to try to become more physically active.[69,70]

Clearly, goals will change from patient to patient. The adolescent patient, who may be overweight but otherwise healthy, should have drastically different goals than the 45-year-old diabetic who is obese and prehypertensive. Although the specific goals will be different, health care providers should be familiar with the guidelines in the goal-setting process. The good news is that the basic guidelines for goal-setting can be easily followed through the MI process. The first step is patient self-assessment, which can be facilitated through MI and agenda-setting. The process continues with goal setting and goal commitment.[70] When setting specific goals to increase

physical activity, the health care provider should assist the patient in creating realistic, but challenging goals. As with goals that are unattainable, those that are not specific or too easy to accomplish often do not provide enough motivation to help the patient continue the behavior.[68–70] If needed, smaller, more attainable objectives may be helpful to build patient self-efficacy.

Through routine follow-up, the health care practitioner should follow the next phase of goal setting, which is to solicit feedback from the patient on progress.[70] If progress is slow, the practitioner may need to readdress the patient's barriers and challenges. It is essential to remember that patients will cycle through stages of behavior change, so just because a patient has begun preparation or action to become more physically active, that does not mean they will continue.[21] Feedback to patients should focus on the accomplishments and rewards of the change to become more physically active. Positively framed communication related to the successes of the patient's behavior change plan will enhance the promotion of self-efficacy and provide increased motivation to sustain the physically active lifestyle.[70]

OTHER COUNSELING STRATEGIES

Although MI holds significant promise for health care providers seeking to increase physical activity among patients, there are many other evidence-based counseling strategies that can be utilized. One such strategy is the Patient-centered Assessment and Counseling for Exercise and Nutrition (PACE). PACE allows for brief physical activity assessment and counseling during routine office visits.[71–75] The process begins with a brief assessment form completed by the patient while waiting to see the health care provider. On the basis of the patient's assessment responses, the health care provider is able to deliver a patient counseling protocol targeted to his or her current level of activity and motivation for change. PACE is designed around the stages of change, allowing the practitioners to deliver stage-specific advice based on the patient's readiness for change.[75] PACE materials and products are available through www.paceproject.org. Specific products included targeted materials for adults and postpartum women.

Alternative strategies, such as telephone counseling, have also proved to be successful with patients. Through the Veterans Life Study, older adults were offered a modified PACE counseling curriculum called *Project Life*.[76,77] This program offered brief baseline counseling on physical activity, whereas continued counseling took place via telephone within subsequent weeks and months. The standard telephone counseling protocol aimed to assess physical activity goals, determine actual physical activity participation, offer support, discuss barriers, address problems, and create new goals for the patient.[77] Monthly automated telephone messages delivered by the health care provider also encouraged patients as they attempted to increase their physical activity levels. Because many health care providers report lack of time is a deterrent to offering physical activity counseling to patients,[78,79] this unique approach of tele-counseling may indeed be an alternative.[77]

Advocacy Efforts for Policy Change

Understanding the basic guidelines for physical activity and knowing how to counsel patients to become more physically active can play a huge role in preventing many of the health problems that the population experiences today. Despite the efforts of health care providers with individual patients, there will still be a need to address the overall lack of physical activity at the population-level through local community, state, or even national advocacy. Practitioners are in the unique position of being influential to both individuals and population; therefore, a practitioner can be a very effective advocate.[80–83]

Health education advocacy is a core responsibility of Certified Health Education Specialists.[84] Although the responsibilities of health educators and health care providers are different, the overall objective of the two professions is the same—to improve the health of the individuals served. To this end, health care providers should also seek to be active in advocacy efforts to increase physical activity at the population level. Change in local or state policy represents a major macro-level social ecological influence on behavior; consequently, it can have a large effect on the population's participation in physical activity. A primary example of policy change impacting health outcomes can be seen in areas that enact smoke-free ordinances.[85–88] As policies prohibiting smoking in public places are implemented, a reduction in the overall number of smokers is reduced. This major change in the environment or ecology of the individual provides a key influence that impacts behavioral choices. Although systematic policy changes promoting physical activity are not as common as tobacco policies, there is some evidence to suggest that making the environment more exercise-friendly tends to increase individuals' participation in physical activity. Table 8.6 indicates areas of policy development for which a health care provider may be able to advocate.

Advocacy is a very involved process that requires a commitment of time, effort, and expertise. The results, however, can be both professionally and personally rewarding. The International Council of Nurses has released the call to advocacy action for health care providers through which the council has identified a 10-step framework describing advocacy participation.[97] These steps are:

1. Overcoming obstacles to action
2. Identifying and drawing attention to an issue

TABLE 8.6	Potential Physical Activity Advocacy Areas for Health Care Providers Outside of Traditional Health Care Settings	
Setting	**Advocacy Needs**	**References**
School health	Increased participation in daily, organized physical education classes	89
	Mandatory completion of health education in K-12 schools	90
	Implementation of walk-to-school programs	91
Community health	Sidewalk and bike lane ordinances targeting increased and improved nonmotorized travel	92 92
	Allocation of public resources for low-cost recreational facilities (city parks, walking trials, etc.)	93, 94
	Improved law enforcement for reduction in crime	
Practitioner education and training	Increased training on physical activity recommendations and guidelines	95, 96
	Formalized education on health promotion strategies and techniques	96

3. Identifying the key people you need to influence
4. Doing your homework on the issue and mapping the potential roles of relevant players
5. Winning the support of key individuals/organizations
6. Collectively identifying goals and objectives and best ways to achieve them
7. Delivering your messages and counteracting the efforts of opposing interest groups
8. Timing interventions and actions for maximum impact
9. Monitoring and evaluating process and impact
10. Building sustainable capacity throughout the process[97]

Practitioners should seek out opportunities with local, state, or national coalitions whose goals include physical activity promotion among the population. The National Coalition for Promoting Physical Activity has established a nationwide physical activity plan for the US.[98] This plan highlights areas in which advocacy is needed, including industry, education, health care, mass media, recreation, public health, transportation, community design, and volunteer organizations. All these areas present excellent opportunities for health care providers to share their expertise in health and lead the charge for policy change to promote better ecological access to physical activity. Other areas of physical activity advocacy can be found at the National Association for Sport and Physical Education's website.[99]

Literature Cited

1. Centers for Disease Control and Prevention. Physical Activity and Health. http://www.cdc.gov/physicalactivity/everyone/health/index.html. Accessed February 29, 2011.
2. Nelson M, Rejeski WJ, Blair SN, et al. Physical activity and public health in older adults: recommendation from the American College of Sports Medicine and the American Heart Association. *Med Sci Sport Exerc*. 2007;39(8):1435–1445.
3. Schnohr P, Scharling H, Jenson JS. Changes in leisure-time physical activity and risk of death: an observational study of 7,000 men and women. *Am J Epidemiol*. 2003;158(7):639–644.
4. Haskell WL, Lee IM, Pate RR, et al. Physical activity and public health: updated recommendation for adults from the American College of Sports Medicine and the American Heart Association. *Med Sci Sport Exerc*. 2007;39(8):1423–1434.
5. Anis NA, Lee RE, Ellerbeck EF, et al. Direct observation of physician counseling on dietary habits and exercise: patient, physician, and office correlates. *Prev Med*. 2004;38(2):198–202.
6. Flocke SA, Kelly R, Highland, J. Initiation of health behavior discussions during primary

care outpatient visits. *Patient Edu Couns.* 2009; 75:214–219.

7. Weidinger KA, Lovegreen SL, Elliot MB, et al. How to make exercise counseling more effective: lessons from rural America. *J Fam Pract.*2008;57(6):394–402.

8. U.S. Department of Health and Human Services. 2008 Physical Activity Guidelines for Americans. http://www.health.gov/paguidelines. Accessed February 29, 2011.

9. Watkinson C, van Sluijs EM, Sutton S, et al. Overestimation of physical activity level is associated with lower BMI: a cross-sectional analysis. *Int J Behav Nutr Phys Act.*2010;7:68.

10. Ronda G, Van Assema P, Brug J. Stages of change, psychological factors and awareness of physical activity levels in The Netherlands. *Health Promot Int.*2001;16:305–314.

11. van Sluijs EMF, Griffin SJ, van Poppel MN. A cross-sectional study of awareness of physical activity: associations with personal, behavioral and psychosocial factors. *Int J Behav Nutr Phys Act.*2007;4:53.

12. Jago R, Anderson CB, Baranowski T, et al. Adolescent patterns of physical activity differences by gender, day, and time of day. *Am J Prev Med.* 2005;28(5):447–452.

13. Caspersen CJ, Pereira MA, Curran KM. Changes in physical activity patterns in the United States, by sex and cross-sectional age. *Med Sci Sports Exerc.* 2000;32(9):1601–1609.

14. Kimm SY, Glynn NW, Kriska AM, et al. Decline in physical activity in black girls and white girls during adolescence. *N Engl J Med.* 2002; 347(10):709–715.

15. U.S. Department of Health and Human Services. Physical Activity Guidelines Advisory Committee Report. http://www.health.gov/PAguidelines/Report. Accessed March 1, 2011.

16. Adachi-Mejia AM, Drake KM, MacKenzie TA, et al. Perceived intrinsic barriers to physical activity among rural mothers. *J Womens Health (Larchmt).* 2010;19 (12):2197–2202.

17. Brown PR, Brown WJ, Miller YD, et al. Perceived constraints and social support for active leisure among mothers with young children. *Leisure Sci.* 2008;23:131–144.

18 Felton GM, Dowda M, Ward DS, et al. Differences in physical activity between black and white girls living in rural and urban areas. *J Sch Health.* 2002;72:250–255.

19. Grubbs L, Carter J. The relationship of perceived benefits and barriers to reported exercise behaviors in college undergraduates. *Fam Community Health.* 2002;25(2):76–84.

20. Tergerson JL, King KA. Doperceived cues, benefits, and barriers to physical activity differ between male and female adolescents? *J Sch Health.* 2002;72(9):374–380.

21. Glanz, K, Rimer, B. *Theory at a glance: a guide for health promotion practice.* Bethesda, MD: National Cancer Institute; 1995.

22. Bronfenbrenner U. Toward an experimental ecology of human development. *Am Psycho.*1977;32:513–531.

23. Bronfenbrenner U. *The Ecology of Human Development.* Cambridge: Harvard University Press; 1979.

24. McLeroy K, Bibeau D, Steckler A, et al. An ecological perspective on health promotion programs. *Health Educ Q.*1988;15(4):351–377.

25. Stokols D. Establishing and maintaining healthy environments. Toward a social ecology of health promotion. *Am Psychol.* 1992;47(1):6–22.

26. Stokols D. Translating social ecological theory into guidelines for community health promotion. *Am J Health Promot.* 1996;10(4): 282–298.

27. Richard L, Potvin L, Kishchuk N, et al. Assessment of the integration of the ecological approach in health promotion programs. *Am J Health Promot.*1996;10(4);318–328.

28. Kok G, Gottlieb NH, Commers M, et al. The ecological approach in health promotion programs: a decade later. *Am J Health Promot.* 2008;22(6):437–442.

29. Williams R, Perko M, Belcher D, et al. Use of social ecology model to address alcohol use among college athletes. *Am J Health Studies.* 2006;21(4):228–237.

30. Williams R, Perko M, Usdan S, et al. Influences on alcohol use among NCAA athletes: application of the social ecology model. *Am J Health Studies.*2008;23(3):151–159.

31. Williams R, Belcher D. Alcohol-related social and personal problems of undergraduate college students [Abstract].*Res Q Exercise Sport.* 2007;78(1):A37.

32. Dwyer J, Needham L, Simpson JR, et al. Parents report intrapersonal, interpersonal, and environmental barriers to supporting healthy eating and physical activity among their preschoolers. *Appl Physiol Nutr Metab.*2008;33.330–340.

33. Bull S, Eakin E, Reeves M, et al. Multi-level support for physical activity and healthy eating. *J Adv Nurs.* 2006;54(5):585–593.

34. Fleury J, Lee SM. The social ecological model and physical activity in African American women. *Am J Commun Psychol.* 2006;37(1–2): 129–140.

35. Tompkins TH, Belza B, Brown MA. Nurse practitioner practice patterns for exercise counseling. *J Am Acad Nurse Pract.* 2009;21:79–86.

36. Dugdill L, Graham R, McNair F. Exercise referral: the public health panacea for physical activity promotion? A critical perspective of exercise referral schemes; their development and evaluation. *Ergonomics.* 2005;48(11–14):1390–1410.

37. Elley R, Kerse N, Arroll B, et al. Effectiveness of counseling patients on physical activity in general practice: cluster randomised controlled trial. *BMJ.* 2003;326(7393):793–800.

38. Walsh J, Swangard D, Davis T, et al. Exercise counseling by primary care physicians in the era of managed care. *Am J Prev Med.* 1999;16(4):307–313.

39. Zimmerman GL, Olsen CG, Bosworth MF. A "stages of change" approach to helping patients change behavior. *Am Fam Physician.* 2000;61(5):1409–1416.

40. World Health Organization. Integrating Prevention into Health Care. http://whqlibdoc.who.int/fact_sheet/2002/FS_172.pdf. Accessed June 21, 2011.

41. Prochaska JO, DiClemente CC, Norcross JC. In search of how people change. Applications to addictive behaviors. *Am Psychol.* 1992;47(9):1102–1114.

42. Prochaska JO, DiClemente CC. The transtheoretical approach. In: Norcross JC, Goldfried MR, ed. *Handbook of Psychotherapy Integration.* 2nd ed. New York, NY: Oxford University Press, 2005. 147–171.

43. Miller WR, Rollnick S. *Motivational Interviewing: preparing people for change.* 2nd ed. New York, NY: Guilford Press, 2002.

44. Miller WR. Motivational interviewing with problem drinkers. *Behav Psychother.* 1983;11:147–172.

45. Britt E, Hudson SM, Blampied, NM. Motivational interviewing in health settings: a review. *Patient Educ Couns.* 2004;53(2):147–155.

46. Stotts AL, DiClementi CC, Dolan-Mullen P. A motivational intervention for resistant pregnant smokers. *Addict Behav.* 2002;27(2):275–292.

47. Valanis B, Lichenstein E, Mulloly JP, et al. Maternal smoking cessation and relapse prevention during health care visits. *Am J Prev Med.* 2001;20(1):1–8.

48. Doherty Y, Roberts S. Motivational interviewing in diabetes practice. *Diabet Med.* 2002;19 Suppl 3:1–6.

49. Rollnick S, Miller WR. What is motivational interviewing? *Behav Cogn Psychol.* 1995;23:325–334.

50. Jones KD, Burckhardt CS, Bennett JA. Motivational interviewing may encourage exercise in persons with fibromyalgia by enhancing self efficacy. *Arthritis Rheum.* 2004;51(5):864–867.

51. Mid-Atlantic Addiction Technology Transfer Center. A definition on motivational interviewing. http://www.motivationalinterview.org/Documents/1%20A%20MI%20Definition%20Principles%20&%20Approach%20V4%20012911.pdf Accessed July 2, 2011.

52. Ang D, Kesavalu R, Lydon JR, et al. Exercise-based motivational interviewing for female patients with fibromyalgia: a case series. *Clin Rheumatol.* 2007;26(11):1843–1849.

53. Brodie DA, Inoue A, Shaw DG. Motivational interviewing to change quality of life for people with chronic heart failure: a randomised controlled trial. *Int J Nurs Stud.* 2008;45(4):489–500.

54. Rhodes RE, Fiala B. Building motivation and sustainability into the prescription and recommendations for physical activity and exercise therapy: the evidence. *Physiotherapy Theo Prac.* 2009;25(5–6):424–441.

55. Schoo A. Motivational interviewing in the prevention and management of chronic disease: improving physical activity and exercise in line with choice theory. *Int J Reality Therapy.* 2008;27(2):26–29.

56. Hardcastle S, Taylor A, Bailey M, et al. A randomised controlled trial on the effectiveness of a primary health care based counselling intervention on physical activity, diet and CHD risk factors. *Patient Educ Couns.* 2008;70(1):31–39.

57. Rash EM. Clinicians' perspectives on motivational interviewing-based brief interventions in college health. *J Am Coll Health.* 2008;57(3):379–380.

58. Rollnick S, Mason P, Butler, C. *Health behavior change: a guide for practitioners.* Edinburgh, Scotland: Churchill Livingstone; 1999.

59. Leach R, Evans W, Williams Jr R, et al. Grand rounds: teen with back pain complicated by obesity. *J Clin Chiropr Pediatr.* 2009;10(2):687–691.

60. Rautalinko E, Lisper HO, Ekehammar B. Reflective listening in counseling: effects of training time and evaluator social skills. *Am J Psychother.* 2007;61(2):191–209.

61. Rose EA, Parfitt G, Williams S. Exercise causality orientations, behavioural regulations for exercise and stage of change for exercise: exploring their relationships. *Psychol Sport Exerc.* 2005;6:399–414.

62. Landry JB, Solmon MA. African American women's self-determination across the stages of change for exercise. *J Sport Exerc Psychol.* 2004;26:457–469.

63. Daley AJ, Duda JL. Self-determination, stage of readiness to change for exercise, and frequency of

physical activity in young people. *Eur J Sport Sci.* 2006;6(4):231–243.

64. Hesse M. The readiness ruler as a measure of readiness to change poly-drug use in drug abusers. *Harm Reduction J.* 2006;3:3CrackauB, Loehrmann I, Zahradnik A, et al. Measuring readiness to change for problematic consumption of prescription drugs: development of an adapted and shortened Readiness to Change Questionnaire. *Addict Res Theory.* 2010;18(1):110–118.

64. Marcus BH, Dubbert PM, Forsyth LH, et al. Physical activity behavior change: issues in adoption and maintenance. *Health Psychol.* 2000;19(1S):32–41.

65. Potter MB, Vu JD, Croughan-Minihane M. Weight management: what patients want from their primary care physicians. *J Fam Pract.* 2001; 50(6):513–518.

66. Locke EA, Latham GP. New directions in goal-setting theory. *Curr Dir Psychol Sci.* 2006;15(5):265–268.

67. Strecher VJ, Seijts GH, Kok GJ, et al. Goal setting as a strategy for health behavior change. *Health Edu Q.*1995;22(2):190–200.

68. Shilts MK, Horowitz M, Townsend MS. Goal setting as a strategy for dietary and physical activity behavior change: a review of the literature. *Am J Health Promot.* 2004;19(2):81–93.

69. Calfas KJ, Long BJ, Sallis JF, et al. A controlled trial of physician counseling to promote the adoption of physical activity. *Prev Med.* 1996;25(3):225–233.

70. Patrick K, Sallis JF, Long B, et al. A new tool for encouraging activity: project PACE. *Physician Sportsmed.* 1994;22(11):45–52.

71. Long BJ, Calfas KJ, Wooten W, et al. A multisite field test of the acceptability of physical activity counseling in primary care: project PACE. *Am J Prev Med.* 1996;12(2):73–81.

72. Calfas KJ, Sallas JF, Zabinski MF, et al. Preliminary evaluation of a multicomponent program for nutrition and physical activity change in primary care: PACE+ for adults. *Prev Med.* 2002;34(2):153–161.

73. Blackburn DG. Establishing an effective framework for physician activity counseling in primary care settings. *Nutr Clin Care.* 2002;5(3): 95–102.

74. Morey MC, Peterson MJ, Pieper CF, et al. Project LIFE—Learning to improve fitness and function in elders: methods, design, and baseline characteristics of randomized trial. *J Rehabil Res Dev.* 2008;45(1):31–42.

75. Morey MC, Peterson MJ, Pieper CF, et al. The veterans learning to improve fitness and function in elders study: a randomized trial of primary care–based physical activity counseling for older men. *J Am Geriatr Soc.* 2009;57(7):1166–1174.

76. Anderson RT, King A, Stewart AL, et al. Physical activity counseling in primary care and patient well-being: do patients benefit? *Ann Behav Med.* 2005;30(2):146–154.

77. Jacobson DM, Strochecker L, Comptom MT, et al. Physical activity counseling in the adult primary care setting: position statement of the American College of Preventive Medicine. *Am J Prev Med.* 2005;29(2):158–162.

78. Williams R, Evans MW, Perko M. Health promotion advocacy: a practitioner's role in prevention of sports injuries. *T Integrative Hlthc.* 2011;2(1):2.1003.

79. Evans MW Jr, Williams RD, Perko M. Public health advocacy and chiropractic: a guide to helping your community reach its health objectives. *J Chiropr Med.* 2008;7(2):71–77.

80. Herbert CP. Physicians and advocacy. *CMAJ.* 2005;173(6):578.

81. Li JT. The physician as advocate. *Mayo Clin Proc.* 1998;73(10):1022–1024.

82. National Commission for Health Education Credentialing. Responsibilities and Competencies of Health Educators. http://www.nchec.org/credentialing/responsibilities. Accessed July 18, 2011.

83. Lee JT, Glantz SA, Millet C. Effect of smoke-free legislation on adult smoking behaviour in England in the 18 months following implementation. *PLoS One.* 2011;6(6):e20933.

84. Wakefield M, Cameron M, Murphy M. Potential for smoke-free policies in social venues to prevent smoking uptake and reduce relapse: a qualitative study. *Health Promot Pract.* 2009;10(1):119–127.

85. Fichtenberg CM, Glantz SA. Effect of smoke-free workplaces on smoking behavior: systematic review. *BMJ.* 2002;325(7357):188.

86. Philpot SJ, Ryan S, Torre L, et al. Effect of smoke-free policies on the behaviour of social smokers. *Tob Control.* 1998;8(3):278–281.

87. Story M, Nanney MS, Schwartz MB. Schools and obesity prevention: creating school environments and policies to promote healthy eating and physical activity. *Milbank Q.* 2009;87(1):71–100.

88. American Cancer Society, American Diabetes Association, American Health Association. Health Education in Schools—The Importance of Establishing Healthy Behaviors in our Nation's Youth. http://www.aahperd.org/aahe/advocacy/positionStatements/upload/statement-ACS-AHA-ADA.pdf. Accessed July 21, 2011.

89. Centers for Disease Control and Prevention. Kids Walk to School. http://www.cdc.gov/nccd-php/dnpa/kidswalk. Accessed July 21, 2011.

90. Librett JJ, Yore MM, Schmid TL. Local ordinances that promote physical activity: a survey of municipal policies. *Am J Public Health.* 2003;93(9):1399–1403.

91. Brown RA, Ottensmann J, Lindsey G, et al. The impact of crime on physical activity: incorporating crime measures in trail use models. http://www.activelivingresearch.org/files/Brown_Context_2007.pdf. Accessed July 21, 2011.

92. Harrison, RA, Gemmell I, Heller RF. The population effect of crime and neighborhood on physical activity: an analysis of 15,461 adults. *J Epidemiol Community Health.* 2007;61(1):34–39.

93. Douglas F, Torrance M, van Teijlingen E, et al. Primary care staff's views and experiences related to routinely advising patients about physical activity. A questionnaire survey. *BMC Public Health.* 2006;6:138.

94. Santiago OJ, Feltz D, Mickus M, et al. Medical student's self-efficacy in physical activity counseling to older adults. *J Sports Exerc Psychol.* 2007;29(Supp):S201.

95. International Council of Nurses. Promoting health: advocacy guide for health professionals. http://www.whpa.org/PPE_Advocacy_Guide.pdf.. Accessed July 21, 2011.

96. National Coalition for Promoting Physical Activity. National Physical Activity Plan. http://www.physicalactivityplan.org/index.php. Accessed July 21, 2011.

97. National Association for Sport and Physical Education. Advocacy toolkit. http://www.aahperd.org/naspe/advocacy/governmentrelations/toolkit.cfm. Accessed July 21, 2011.

CHAPTER 9

Nutrition for Prevention and Health Promotion

Daniel Redwood

Diet and nutrition play a central role in preventing disease and restoring health. The oft-quoted phrase, "An ounce of prevention is worth a pound of cure," meshes perfectly with contemporary health sciences research. In general, nutritional approaches that help to prevent a disease are also appropriate when seeking to arrest or reverse its course. This chapter focuses on prevention and health promotion rather than targeted nutritional treatment of diagnosed disease processes.

BECOMING PART OF THE SOLUTION

Popular culture steadily bombards us with around-the-clock messaging about foods and beverages. Little of this is consistent with nutritional research; most is no more than corporate marketing. Television programming in the United States is awash in ads for foods and beverages that promote illness and obesity, alongside ads for the pharmaceuticals used to treat the ailments caused by these foods and beverages. The absence of any significant countervailing message urging viewers to seek out the vegetables, fruits, and other whole foods known to be cornerstones of good health is more than a disgrace—it is a national tragedy. Most people believe what they are repeatedly told, especially when exposure to these ideas begins at an age when their capacity for critical thinking has not yet developed and matured.

When we share accurate nutrition information with our patients and give them the tools to choose a well-rounded, health-affirming diet, we become part of the solution to this public health crisis.

NATURAL HEALTH, NATURAL DIET: AN ECOLOGIC PERSPECTIVE

The most fundamental principle of the natural healing arts is that human beings should strive to live in harmony with nature. For almost the entire history of the human race, people in hunter–gatherer and agricultural societies alike have eaten diets primarily based on whole foods, locally grown, processed minimally if at all, and devoid of industrial chemicals. This is our natural diet. Long-term human health patterns reflect a process of coevolution with our environment; the foods and beverages we consume each day represent our most intimate interchange with that environment. From an epigenetic perspective, we are feeding not only ourselves but also future generations.[1]

The great lesson we have learned from the science of ecology is that components of natural systems are richly interactive, with cause-and-effect relationships moving simultaneously in all directions in a complex network of multiple feedback loops. This has wide-ranging implications. The key application for the healing arts—by no means fully appreciated and integrated as yet—is a growing and probably irreversible loss of legitimacy for single-source causation as a fundamental organizing principle in the health sciences.

This is especially important in the nutritional arena. Prescribing a single nutrient to cure a disease, mitigate a symptom, or suppress pain is, at its root, a pharmaceutical approach. It can certainly be helpful in some cases, but if this becomes our primary focus, we risk losing sight of the larger picture. Over time, encouraging our patients to focus on the therapeutic role of isolated nutrients (i.e., taking a certain number of milligrams of a particular vitamin or fatty acid) confuses more than it clarifies; it also fosters dependency on experts (ourselves and others) to explain the complex mathematics of nutritional science.

Instead, we need to direct our attention to the patient's whole diet. Teaching patients to distinguish between helpful and harmful foods, and teaching them to create meals that are both health-affirming and enjoyable serves them far better in the long run.

FOUNDATIONS OF A HEALTHY DIET

Changes in the Establishment Consensus

Until the 20th century, a broad consensus in the medical establishment held that in developed nations where starvation and near-starvation had been almost completely eliminated, nutrition played a minimal role in the causation of disease and almost no role in its treatment, except for a small number of specific applications in conditions such as celiac disease, hypertension, and diabetes. In that era, patients with cancer or cardiovascular disease, for example, were almost never asked to change their diets and the population as a whole was not urged to eat certain foods and avoid others as a means of preventing illness.

In the past few decades, nutrition research has expanded exponentially, bringing with it an evolving perspective on the importance of diet. To give just one indicator of the scale of this change, in 1981 the *Journal of the National Cancer Institute* published a landmark paper by Doll and Peto,[2] which found that nutrition plays a role in the causation in 35% to 60% of cancer cases. Soon after that, NCI began to promote dietary guidance for minimizing cancer risk, focused on eating substantial quantities of vegetables, fruits, and whole grains while minimizing intake of fatty meats and full-fat dairy products. All government health agencies and major nonprofit health advocacy groups now recognize that diet is a critical component of strategies for disease prevention and health promotion.

Areas of Agreement, Areas of Controversy

There is now essentially universal consensus on the importance of some foods and food groups in preventing disease and maintaining health, along with ongoing disagreement about the pluses and minuses of other foods and food groups.

Vegetables and fruits generate virtually no controversy, other than debates on how to effectively convince people to eat a combined total of five or more servings per day.[3] *Whole grains and legumes* (beans, peas, and lentils) are also widely judged to be highly beneficial by the nutrition research and nutrition policy communities—including the Surgeon General,[4] American Dietetic Association,[5] Harvard School of Public Health,[6] American Heart Association (AHA),[7] American Diabetes Association,[8] American Cancer Society,[9,10] and a wide range of other conventional

and alternative sources. Inaccurate claims that whole grains are inflammatory and that soy foods increase the risk of breast cancer will be addressed later in this chapter.

Non-processed meats, eggs, and fish are also recommended as dietary components by the major pillars of the health care establishment—the USDA, NIH, Surgeon General, and the major health advocacy organizations mentioned above. Official recommendations about these animal-derived foods are in many cases coupled with advice to keep intake *at or below* a specified amount. In contrast, recommendations on vegetables, fruits, whole grains, and legumes generally call for intake *at or above* a certain level. Diets that do not include meats, fish, or eggs are also widely acknowledged to be a healthy option, as expressed by the American Dietetic Association's policy statement, which concluded that "well-planned vegetarian diets are appropriate for individuals during all stages of the life cycle, including pregnancy, lactation, infancy, childhood, and adolescence, and for athletes."[11]

In many ways, dairy products are in a class by themselves. People in all Western nations have been taught that milk, cheese, and other dairy products are essential to build and maintain healthy bones, and dairy remains the most common source of dietary calcium in Western nations. However, in recent years, a growing body of high-quality research[12,13] has raised questions about the credibility of such claims, leading major figures in the nutritional science world, most notably Walter Willett of the Harvard School of Public Health, to call for reconsideration of the role of dairy in bone health[14] and health in general.[15] This is explored in greater depth later in this chapter.

Foods and Drinks to Minimize or Exclude

To help guide needed dietary changes, whether on an individual or population-wide basis, it is important to focus not only on foods that should be included, but also on those that should be minimized or excluded. Given current American dietary patterns, perhaps the most important nutritional advice we can give our patients is to sharply limit intake of high-calorie, low-nutrient foods. For many people, these comprise a majority of food and beverage intakes. Arguably, the worst offenders are soda pop and other sweet drinks (accurately described as "liquid candy"),[16] processed meats, and foods containing hydrogenated oils, but the list of foods and drinks delivering excessive quantities of sugars, fats, and salt is virtually endless.

Aside from the direct damage inflicted by these junk foods, they cause significant further harm by displacing healthy foods. Someone who has just filled up on a double burger with fries and a large cola or milkshake is not going to be hungry for vegetables, fruits, beans, and whole grains. With some of our patients, this is the point at which we must begin.

USDA Dietary Guidelines: Plate Replaces Pyramid

In 2011, the U.S. Department of Agriculture discontinued its Food Pyramid, replacing it with MyPlate (www.choosemyplate.gov). Half of MyPlate (and therefore half of recommended daily food intake) is devoted to vegetables and fruits. Slightly more than a quarter of the plate is for grains, with the remainder allotted to a more confusing category labeled "proteins," which includes meats and beans but not dairy products. A small circle representing the dairy group (which includes animal milk products as well as soy milk) appears beside the plate (Fig. 9.1).

The most dramatic immediate impression created by the MyPlate icon is that vegetables and fruits clearly and visibly fill 50% of the plate. Also noteworthy is that meats and other proteins account for less than a quarter of the plate, since it is not uncommon for an actual American dinner plate to have the majority of its space occupied by a meat entree. Currently, most Americans fall far short of the goals advanced by USDA and MyPlate.

Harvard School of Public Health: Healthy Eating Plate

In response to the USDA MyPlate, the Harvard School of Public Health produced an amended version, the Healthy Eating Plate (Fig. 9.2), with (1) water replacing dairy as the primary recommended beverage; (2) "whole grains" replacing "grains"; (3) "healthy protein" replacing "protein," and (4) an additional category, healthy oils, such as olive and canola. Perhaps most importantly, the Healthy Eating Plate illustration includes brief written explanations that clarify issues about the various food groups that the USDA MyPlate leaves largely undefined.

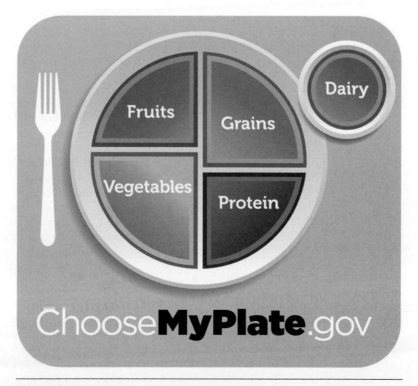

Figure 9.1. My Plate.

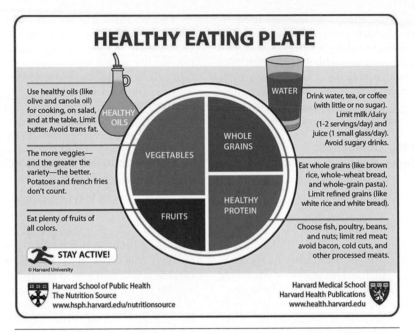

Figure 9.2. Healthy Eating Plate. (Copyright © 2011 Harvard University. For more information about The Healthy Eating Plate, please see The Nutrition Source, Department of Nutrition, Harvard School of Public Health, http://www.hsph.harvard.edu/nutritionsource/ and Harvard Health Publications, www.health.harvard.edu.)

MAJOR FOOD GROUPS

Vegetables and Fruits

The health value of vegetables and fruits is undisputed; all evidence-based dietary guidelines urge people to have a minimum of five servings per day. Patients should be encouraged not only to meet or exceed the 5-per-day standard but also to choose a variety of different vegetables and fruits (thus providing a wide range of vitamins and other nutrients), while also including some of the foods known to be most nutrient-dense. For example, dark green leafy vegetables (e.g., kale, collards, and broccoli) are strong sources of calcium, as are members of the bean family. "Greens and beans" offers the best nondairy dietary strategy for achieving sufficient calcium intake. Among fruits, some berries (e.g., blueberries, raspberries, and cranberries) are extraordinarily high in antioxidants. Diets that include a wide range of fruits and vegetables are far better than those where a few foods are eaten repeatedly and exclusively.

While the sweetness of fresh fruits appeals to most people, vegetables can offer a greater challenge. Many people form a negative impression of the entire vegetable kingdom early in life as a result of unpleasant experiences with, for example, severely overcooked broccoli or spinach. For these individuals and others, it is important to emphasize the need to find ways to make vegetables not just tolerable but enjoyable. People who see eating vegetables as an unpleasant chore are far less likely to sustain a commitment to healthy eating. Spices and sauces can play a key role in enhancing the taste of vegetables. If someone loves marinara sauce, teriyaki sauce, curry, ginger, hot chili peppers, parsley, sage, rosemary, or thyme, alone or combined, he or she should be encouraged to use these to add familiar and enjoyable tastes to unfamiliar vegetables.

Economic Issues

From the standpoint of clinicians seeking to guide patients toward healthier dietary patterns, it is important to consider that, in addition to the lack of knowledge and/or willpower that keep many people from eating adequate quantities of nutrient-rich foods, economic forces add to the difficulties experienced by many at the lower end of the economic ladder. "Food deserts," inner city neighborhoods where no food markets are accessible to people lacking a car, offer additional challenges to those already challenged economically. Moreover, in times of economic downturn or high unemployment, many in the struggling middle class are forced to limit expenses, which may include cutbacks on food purchases. Health professionals advising such patients must be sensitive to these social influences.

Further aggravating the situation in the US, government policies tilt heavily toward the meat and dairy industries, with 63% of government agricultural subsidies going to growers of those foods versus less than 1% for fruits and vegetables.[17] These USDA subsidy policies directly undercut USDA health policies, artificially depressing the price of meat and dairy in comparison to fruits and vegetables.

Cereal Grains

A broad, deep, and sustained consensus in the field of evidence-based nutrition recommends the inclusion of whole grains as an integral part of a healthy diet. These whole foods are cost-effective staples that can help anchor the nutritional component of a healthy lifestyle.[18] Whole grains, with the bran and germ intact, are nutritionally superior to refined grains. For example, a slice of commercially prepared white bread has 66 calories, 1.9 grams of protein, and 0.6 grams of fiber. In contrast, a slice of whole wheat bread has 69 calories and provides 3.6 grams of protein and 1.9 grams of fiber.[19]

ARE WHOLE GRAINS INFLAMMATORY?

Attacks against whole grains can be found on popular websites serving the alternative health[20,21] community, based in large part on unsubstantiated claims that both whole and refined cereal grains cause or accelerate inflammation in the body. Sometimes, this assertion is presented as established fact,[21] with no indication to readers of its highly controversial nature. Since inflammation is known to be a key factor in diseases ranging from cardiovascular disease to diabetes to low back pain, this is a serious charge that merits clear-minded evaluation.

For anyone wishing to ascertain whether whole grains are inflammatory, a search of PubMed (a National Library of Medicine database) is highly recommended. Using the search terms "inflammation" and "whole grains," a PubMed search (June 14, 2011) yielded 27 references.[22–48]

None of these 27 studies indicated that whole grains are inflammatory; nearly all reported a negative association between whole grain intake and markers of inflammation. That is, current evidence strongly suggests that whole grains have an anti-inflammatory effect, albeit a mild one.

The evidence on *refined grains*, which have had much of their fiber and other nutrients removed (including vitamin E and B-complex), is quite the opposite. Refined grains are pro-inflammatory and associated with increased risk for a wide range of diseases.[22,24,25,30,38,39,41,43,45,49] Intake of refined flour products (white or "wheat" bread, white pasta, etc.) should be avoided whenever possible. Currently, the vast majority of Americans consume grains in the form of white flour products. Federal health guidelines currently recommend that whole grains be preferred over refined grains, with at least 50% of grains eaten in the whole grain form. This is a worthwhile goal; in terms of positive health impact, however, a goal closer to 100% would be even better. Currently, less than 5% of Americans consume the minimum recommended amount of whole grains, which is about three servings per day.[50]

Anyone with celiac disease, gluten intolerance, or an allergy or sensitivity to a particular cereal grain, such as wheat or corn, should avoid the offending food.

Beans and Soy

Beans provide an excellent source of dietary protein, including the amino acid lysine, of which most grains supply only minimal amounts. The amino acids in grains and beans are complementary, together forming a complete protein. Beans are low in calories and high in fiber, a desirable combination.

There is widespread agreement regarding the health value of beans and legumes, which are universally recommended by federal health agencies such as NIH and the Surgeon General's office, as well as all establishment health advocacy organizations such as the American Diabetes Association and AHA. But as with whole grains, there is a persistent, Internet-based attack campaign against beans, particularly soybeans. The most serious attacks allege that soy foods may (1) cause or aggravate breast cancer and (2) exert feminizing effects on men. The inaccuracies propagated in these attacks merit thorough examination, because they have convinced many people to avoid soy, which is the strongest source of nonanimal-based protein.

Longstanding concerns about soy and breast cancer may be nearing resolution, with soy shown to be protective or neutral rather than harmful for women, not only for primary prevention but even for women being treated for breast cancer.[51] Research on this subject is accelerating. Most significantly, a large study[51] by Guha and colleagues followed women with breast cancer undergoing treatment with the chemotherapy agent, tamoxifen. These investigators found that patients whose diets were highest in daidzein, a soy isoflavone, had approximately a 60% reduction in breast cancer recurrence compared to those eating the lowest quantities of soy.

Regarding feminizing effects in men, these occur only with intake of quantities of soy far in excess of usual use, as in the highly publicized case of a Texas man who drank *three quarts of soymilk per day* for many months, during which time his beard growth slowed, he lost hair from his arms, developed breasts, and generally displayed a wide range of feminized characteristics.[52,53] Men whose intake of soy foods is moderate (commonly defined as three servings or less per day) do not experience these disturbing changes. Instead, they benefit from the wide range of nutrients (including protein and fiber) present in soy foods.

SOY AND CANCER PREVENTION

Four major epidemiologic studies have shown that when eaten regularly by girls in childhood and adolescence, soy foods are protective against the development of breast cancer later in life. Even one serving of soy food per day was associated with 25% to 45% reduction of breast cancer. Women who start eating soy later in life do not appear to attain the breast cancer prevention benefit seen among those who ate soy foods in childhood and adolescence.

An American Cancer Society panel published guidelines on nutrition and physical activity for cancer prevention in 2006, which directly addressed the health effects of soy[9]:

"Soy-derived foods are an excellent source of protein and a good alternative to meat. Soy contains several phytochemicals, some of which have weak estrogenic activity and appear to protect against hormone-dependent cancers in animal studies. Presently, there are limited data to support a potential beneficial effect of soy supplements on reducing cancer risk.[54] Furthermore, adverse effects of high doses of soy supplements on the risk of estrogen-responsive cancers, such as breast or endometrial cancer, are possible."[55]

As with other foods and nutrients, clinicians should not assume that soy supplements (extracts or isolates) have effects equivalent to soy foods such as tofu, tempeh, or soymilk.

SOY AND PROSTATE CANCER PREVENTION

An informed consensus that soy helps prevent prostate cancer has emerged among the scientists who closely study the issue. A meta-analysis conducted by Yan and Spitznagel,[56] published in the *American Journal of Clinical Nutrition,* concluded that consumption of soy foods was strongly associated with a lowered risk for prostate cancer.

SOY AND PREVENTION OF CARDIOVASCULAR DISEASE

Since 1995, when three *New England Journal of Medicine* articles showed improvement in cardiovascular markers from eating soy foods,[57-59] including significant decreases in total cholesterol, LDL cholesterol, and triglycerides, the Food and Drug Administration (FDA) has permitted foods containing soy protein to advertise their heart-healthy qualities. Foods that may be eligible for the health claim include soy beverages, tofu, tempeh, and soy-based meat alternatives.

Foods containing soy qualified (and still qualify) for this nutrition claim because the FDA determined that sufficient research justified the claim. However, as further research has emerged, the evidence for these specific cardiovascular claims has weakened. In 2006, a panel representing the AHA Nutrition Committee published a report[60] summarizing new research, which concluded that, "isolated soy protein with isoflavones compared with milk or other proteins decreased LDL cholesterol concentrations in most studies; the average effect was approximately 3%. This reduction is very small ... no benefit is evident on HDL cholesterol, triglycerides, lipoprotein(a), or blood pressure. Thus, the direct cardiovascular health benefit of soy protein or of isoflavone supplements is minimal at best."

The AHA panel nonetheless spoke quite positively about soy as a food, noting "many soy products should be beneficial to cardiovascular and overall health because of their high content of polyunsaturated fats, fiber, vitamins, and minerals and low content of saturated fat." However, they advised against use of soy isoflavone supplements.

Foods, Not Drugs

Foods, including soy, should be considered in the context of the patient's overall diet and lifestyle, not as a singular means to prevent or treat a particular disease. In other words, they should be seen as foods, not drugs. Soy, whole grains, and other healthy foods can be appreciated as sources of valuable nutrients and as potential replacements for less healthy foods. Neither doctors nor patients should see these as cures or guaranteed means of prevention for high cholesterol, coronary heart disease, prostate cancer, or any of the other health issues to which they have been favorably linked.

Dairy

People growing up in the United States have been taught since childhood that bones are primarily made of calcium, that the best dietary sources of calcium are milk and other dairy products, and that consuming these in substantial amounts on a daily basis is necessary to build strong bones. Are these claims and recommendations accurate?

Both facts and context are essential to understand the relationship of dairy, calcium, and bone health. First, dairy products contain substantial amounts of calcium (300 mg in a cup of milk or yogurt, 200 mg in an average serving of cheese). Second, it is true that the mineral content of bone is mainly comprised of calcium (along with phosphorus and other minerals). Third, there is substantial documentation that building up sufficient bone mass in one's early years provides crucial insurance against bone loss in later years.

DOES HIGH CALCIUM INTAKE LEAD TO STRONG BONES?

Putting these facts together, it seems logical to assume that people who consume large amounts of calcium (from dairy products, supplements, or other sources) from childhood onward will have the best bone strength and in later years enjoy the greatest protection against osteoporosis-related fractures. *Research has consistently shown this to be untrue.*

People in nations with highest dairy and calcium intakes have the highest rates of osteoporosis-related fractures, not the lowest. This information has been available in scholarly nutrition research journals since at least the mid-1980s,[61] and recent studies[12] confirm the fundamental point. However, these epidemiologic studies may not fully account for possible confounding factors, such as the fact that most societies with high dairy intake also have high meat intake, and that in many cases this is combined with a sedentary lifestyle. But at the very least, such data demonstrates that no one should count on high dairy or calcium intakes (above a required minimum) to develop or maintain adequate bone density.[62]

EXTRAORDINARY EVIDENCE

As noted in the Harvard Medical School newsletter, HEALTH beat, in 2008[15]:

"For years, high calcium intake has been portrayed as one of the best things you can do to prevent osteoporosis and related fractures. But when researchers started to crunch the data from large, prospective studies that followed people for many years, the benefits weren't so clear-cut. These findings led to randomized trials of calcium to test what effect it might have on fracture rates."

"The tide started to turn in 2005 when results from two British studies showed that calcium didn't prevent fractures—even when taken in combination with vitamin D. The next year, results from a large American trial, the Women's Health Initiative, showed that postmenopausal women who took a calcium–vitamin D combination were no less likely to break a hip than women who took a placebo pill, although the density of their hip bones increased slightly. In 2007, a Swiss and American team, including some researchers from Harvard, reported the results of a meta-analysis of over a dozen studies of calcium. They found no connection between high calcium intake, from either food or pills, and lower hip fracture risk. In fact, when they limited their analysis to four randomized clinical trials with separate results for hip fractures, they found that extra calcium *increased* the risk."

This article went on to note "real drawbacks to overdoing calcium, especially if dairy foods are the source," specifically noting "studies linking high consumption of dairy products to ovarian and prostate cancer ... particularly strong for metastatic and fatal prostate cancer."

THEN WHAT DOES BUILD STRONG BONES?

If calcium intake above a needed minimum (approximately 750 mg/day) is not helpful for building and maintaining bone density,[62] what is the solution? The answer appears to be twofold: weight-bearing exercise and Vitamin D

TABLE 9.1	Approximate Protein Content in One Serving of Selected Foods	
Lean beef (4 oz)		32 g
Pork roast (4 oz)		28 g
Boneless cooked chicken (4 oz)		36 g
Hot dog		7 g
Salmon (3 oz)		28 g
Turkey (4 oz)		36 g
Whole egg		6 g
Milk (1 cup)		8 g
Soymilk (1 cup)		8 g
Low fat yogurt (1 cup)		12 g
Frozen yogurt (1/2 cup)		2.5 g
Cottage cheese (1/2 cup)		14 g
Tofu (8 oz)		9 g
Tempeh (4 oz)		18 g
Peanut butter (2T)		8 g
Beans (1/2 cup)		8 g
Peanuts (1/2 cup)		19 g
Almonds (1/2 cup)		14 g
Sunflower seeds (1/2 cup)		13 g
Whole grain bread (one 1-oz slice)		4 g
Broccoli (1 cup)		5 g
Mushrooms (1 cup)		3 g
Brown rice (1 cup)		5 g
Pasta (1 cup)		6 g

(from sunshine or supplements). An excellent summary of research on this subject, focused primarily on building healthy bones in youth, appeared in *Pediatrics*.[13] The take-home message is: Encouraging children and adolescents to enjoy active play outdoors (exercise plus sunshine vitamin D) is more important than having them drink milk or consume other dairy products, as long as minimum calcium requirements are met.

Meats

Historically, most human societies have consumed meat while some have not. Meats provide the most concentrated form of dietary protein (approximately 30 grams per 4-oz serving), along with other nutrients such as zinc and vitamin B_{12}. Because all of us have received repeated messages throughout our lives (from family members, doctors, and advertisements) warning against protein deficiency, meats of all kinds are seen by many as required dietary components.

To determine the accuracy of such a message, the key initial question is: How much protein do humans need? According to the World Health Organization, the average-sized man requires 56 grams of protein per day and the average-sized woman needs 48 grams per day (see Table 9.1).[63] These requirements can be readily attained through diets with or without meat. Eating meat is a personal choice, not a physical necessity.

In affluent nations, health problems are more likely to arise from having too much meat than too little. Eaten in substantial quantities on a regular basis, the fat content of meats is a major contributor to weight gain. Even lean cuts of meat generally approach 30% of calories from fat. Moreover, the vast majority of meat in beef- and chicken-eating nations such as the United States is not eaten in a lean form; hamburgers and fried chicken have become international symbols of the American way of life. Fast-food outlets, at which fried foods are the most popular fare, are virtually ubiquitous.

Moreover, except for meat raised on organic farms, routine use of antibiotics and growth hormones may bring added risks. Animal agriculture has been clearly identified as a key contributor to the development of antibiotic-resistant microbes.[64] The science regarding adverse effects of growth hormone is less clear. The United States and Canada have long supported widespread use of hormones to accelerate the growth of animals used for food, while the European Union has resisted such efforts, including lengthy court battles to allow its member nations to reject imports of North American meats grown with hormones.[65] On an individual basis, for both men and women, it is possible that the addition of such exogenous hormones to one's system may also have adverse consequences, although the FDA currently deems these safe.[66]

PROCESSED MEATS

Processed meats (bacon, ham, sausage, bologna, salami, corned beef, etc.) are widely agreed to be the most unhealthy type of meat, with their nitrate and nitrosamine content providing a plausible mechanism for evidence indicating an increased risk for cancers of the gastrointestinal tract, particularly the colon.[67] A systematic review found an association between consumption of processed meats and higher incidence of coronary heart disease and diabetes mellitus.[68] Increased risk of stroke has also been documented.[69,70]

RED MEAT

Frequent consumption of red meat may pose health risks. It has been associated with increased risk of cancers of the distal colon,[71] though some studies have found evidence of this association to be weak.[72,73] Red meat has also been associated with cancers of the lung,[74,75] breast,[76] liver,[75] and esophagus,[75] although not all studies have found such associations.[77,78] Of additional concern is the production of carcinogenic mutagens such as the heterocyclic amine PhIP, when red meat is cooked at high temperatures, as in grilling. This has been specifically linked to an elevated risk of developing advanced prostate cancer.[79]

POULTRY

Like other meats, poultry foods are high in protein. Chicken and turkey are sometimes eaten in preference to red meat based on the assumption that poultry represents a healthier choice. Depending on how the meats are prepared, this may or may not be true. For example, research at the National Cancer Institute found that grilling chicken results in substantially higher levels of the carcinogen PhIP (480 nanograms per gram) than is the case for red meat (30 nanograms per gram), 15-fold difference.[80] These effects can be partially mitigated by marination in herbs.[81] The percentage of calories from fat for chicken, although generally lower than for beef, rises substantially if the chicken is fried, deep fried, or basted with butter or oil. Available evidence suggests that for omnivores, poultry should be used in moderation and cooked at relatively low temperatures, preferably in the presence of moisture.[82]

FISH

Fish are a source of protein and omega-3 fatty acids. While most of the fat in fish is not in the omega-3 form, fish oil has significant anti-inflammatory effects. Recommendations from the NIH, Surgeon General, and many others endorse including fish as part of a diet that also emphasizes vegetables, fruits, and whole grains.

Fish can contain significant levels of mercury from industrial pollution of the water in which they swim; hence, the US federal government for many years has recommended that pregnant women and young children limit their consumption of fish for health reasons. Guidelines to this effect were jointly endorsed by the FDA and the Environmental Protection Agency (EPA).[83] However, the two agencies were at loggerheads, to the point of holding competing press conferences on the same day, with the FDA arguing that the health benefits of eating fish outweigh the potential ill effects of mercury while the EPA attacked the FDA opinion as "scientifically flawed and inadequate."[84] It is likely that debate on the benefits and risks of fish consumption will continue for the foreseeable future.

Sugar and Carbohydrates

The carbohydrate content of whole foods—fruits, vegetables, grains, and tubers—has provided the majority of energy (calories) in human diets throughout history. The human appetite for carbohydrates became a problem only when technological advances permitted a high degree of food processing, so that key nutrients (fiber, vitamins, and minerals) could be stripped away with relative ease, rendering such foods calorie-rich but nutrient-poor. Highly industrialized societies have developed food processing to the point where processed foods (or, in the words of food writer, Michael Pollan, "edible food-like substances") are now so widely available that they have replaced whole foods as the majority of the diet for hundreds of millions of people.

Although processed foods as a group are best minimized or avoided, for clinicians discussing diet and nutrition with patients, it is often necessary to decide which specific first steps should be given the highest priority. Consuming five or more servings of fruits and vegetables each day should certainly be high on this list, but a good case can be made that the single most important recommendation should be to sharply limit intake of refined carbohydrates, particularly sugar in all its guises.

TABLE 9.2	Sweeteners Used in Foods
Aspartame—marketed as NutraSweet (artificial, 0 cal)	
Acesulfame potassium (acesulfame-K)/ E950—marketed as Sunett/Sweet One (artificial, 0 cal)	
Brown sugar	
Corn sweetener	
Corn syrup or corn syrup solids	
Dehydrated cane juice	
Dextrin	
Dextrose	
Evaporated cane juice	
Fructose	
Fruit juice concentrate	
Glucose	
High-fructose corn syrup	
Honey	
Invert sugar (golden syrup)	
Lactose	
Maltodextrin	
Malt syrup	
Maltose	
Mannitol (2.6 cal)	
Maple syrup	
Molasses	
Neotame (artificial, 0 cal)	
Raw sugar	
Rice syrup	
Saccharin (artificial, 0 cal)	
Saccharose	
Sucralose—marketed as Splenda (artificial, 0 cal)	
Sucrose	
Sugar	
Sorbitol (2.6 cal)	
Sorghum or sorghum syrup	
Syrup	
Treacle	
Turbinado sugar	
Xylose	

Processed food companies understand all too well that public awareness about the damaging effects of sugar has been significantly raised over the past generation. In response, these corporations have found ways to use multiple forms of refined carbohydrates as sweeteners (see Table 9.2). Because ingredients are listed in order of weight on packaged foods in the United States, this sleight-of-hand allows food companies to divide a food product's sweeteners into several different categories, thus avoiding the economic challenge of marketing a product where sugar or high-fructose corn syrup appears first or second on the list.

SPECIAL ISSUES IN NUTRITION

Obesity and Weight Loss

As recently as 1991, no state in the US had an adult obesity rate (>30 BMI) higher than 15%. By 2011, 38 of 50 states had obesity rates higher than 25%, with 12 states having more than 30% of adults classified as obese. All but one of these states are in the South, led by Mississippi at 34.4%.[85] These statistics do not include people who are overweight but not obese. The combined percentage of overweight plus obese individuals is now approaching 70% of the nation's adult population. The health consequences of these worsening trends are widely understood to be disastrous.

Though the weight loss industry publicizes its individual success stories (some of which are genuinely inspiring), anti-obesity efforts have been a profound failure on a population basis. Changing people's eating habits involves confronting the complex interplay between deeply encoded appetites for sweets and fats that originally evolved to avoid starvation, family eating patterns learned in childhood, and an advertising industry highly skilled at persuading people to continue their destructive dietary habits.

For clinicians seeking to help overweight patients change their diets for the better, the best advice is to encourage the kind of healthy diet described earlier in this chapter. Patients should be urged to emphasize whole foods and minimize junk foods such as refined carbohydrates and fats, while keeping overall fat and calorie intake at reasonable levels. The National Institutes of Health recommends that weight loss goals reflect a gradual but persistent approach within these parameters: (1) reduce body weight by about 10%, an amount that reduces obesity-related risk factors; (2) a reasonable time for the 10% reduction in body weight would be over 6 months, with a weight loss of one to two pounds per week; (3) with success, and if warranted, further weight loss can be attempted. In addition to dietary changes, people trying to lose weight also need to increase their amounts of aerobic exercise.

Vegetarian and Vegan Diets

Vegetarian diets are those that include no meats of any kind but may include dairy products and/or eggs. Vegan diets are vegetarian diets that include no animal-derived products at all.

People choose plant-based diets for three main reasons:

(1) Ethical—to refrain from contributing to unnecessary animal suffering and slaughter
(2) Health—to minimize the risk of illnesses such as cardiovascular disease, cancer, and diabetes
(3) Environmental—because animal agriculture contributes to land degradation, pollution of air and water, depletion of aquifers and other water resources, and loss of biodiversity. In addition, animal agriculture produces more greenhouse gases than all motor vehicles (cars, trucks, planes) combined, according to a 2006 report, Livestock's Long Shadow, by the Food and Agriculture Organization of the United Nations.[86]

As mentioned earlier, a 2009 American Dietetic Association policy statement recognizes the health benefits of well-planned vegetarian and vegan diets. In addition, the two most significant natural health breakthroughs of our era involved randomized trials using such diets. The first was the pioneering research by Dean Ornish and colleagues proving that heart disease can be reversed (something previously thought to be impossible) through a combination of a very low-fat whole foods vegetarian diet, exercise (yoga and walking), meditation, and community support groups.[87–113] The second was the NIH-funded research by Neal Barnard and colleagues that showed a very low-fat whole foods vegan diet to be more effective than the American Diabetes Association diet in reversing diabetes.[114–123] These whole foods, low-fat, plant-based diets are also applicable for prevention of the illnesses they have been proven to effectively treat.

Organic Foods

Since passage of the Organic Foods Production Act of 1990, the U.S. Department of Agriculture has set standards for organic foods, certifying food products grown without the use of synthetic pesticides and fertilizers, genetic engineering, antibiotics, synthetic growth hormones, sewage sludge, and irradiation, and processed without adding artificial flavors, colors, and preservatives. For animal products, the "certified organic" label also means that the animal received no antibiotics or hormones and was given organic feed containing no animal by-products.

GIVING BACK TO THE LAND AND THE LIMITS OF PETROLEUM

The organic movement is based on the environmental ethic of sustainability—of giving back to the land rather than depleting its inherited riches year after year. With proper organic stewardship, land grows more fertile over time from the nutrients returned to it. This is the most natural approach and has great appeal for many people who are drawn to natural health care approaches.[124]

Virtually all agriculture was practiced organically until 20th century, when the invention of petroleum-based industrial chemicals allowed increased crop yields and insect eradication, holding forth the promise that such changes could continue indefinitely. This was a false promise. Our descendants in the post-oil era (likely before the end of this century) will almost certainly look back on the dominant ethos of our time as breathtakingly short-sighted. In the long arc of history, petrochemical agriculture will have been but a brief moment, with short-term benefits for some of those alive at the time and long-term damage for those born later. Climate change, water shortages, and spreading desertification in some of the world's most agriculturally productive areas will be among its lasting legacies, as will ecological disaster zones from the Aral Sea to the Gulf of Mexico. Nature will heal, but not quickly.

ARE ORGANIC FOODS MORE NUTRITIOUS? IS THAT THE MAIN QUESTION?

From an environmental standpoint, organic agriculture is an unalloyed good, preserving the balance of nature in numerous ways. From a health standpoint, there are also significant benefits. The health benefits from avoiding toxic chemicals are clear and growing clearer; however, the nutritive value of organic vis-à-vis conventional food remains controversial.

It may or may not be legitimate to claim that organic foods are more nutritious than those grown conventionally. A 2010 systematic review[125] published in the *American Journal of Clinical Nutrition* concluded that currently available research provides insufficient support for such claims. On the other hand, some studies[126,127] indicate higher nutrient levels in organically raised foods. At this time, a balanced reading of the evidence indicates that this question is unresolved.

PETROCHEMICALS AND THE NERVOUS SYSTEM

Whatever the outcome of the nutrition debate, foods grown on certified organic farms are known to contain far lower levels of pesticides, herbicides, and fungicides—the weaponry of industrial agriculture. Research on specific toxic effects of these chemicals is gradually accumulating, though the interactions among them pose too complex a problem for researchers to adequately address. To put this in context, consider that over 350 chemicals have been identified in human breast milk, from pesticides to flame retardants to gasoline additives to rocket fuel. There is no practical way to study the interactions among these chemicals in vivo. The effects on children and their mothers are largely unknown but certainly not beneficial. In a very real sense, we and our descendants are the subjects of a large-scale biochemistry experiment.

Recently, more specifics on neurologic and other effects of agricultural petrochemicals have emerged, including cognitive effects potentially leading toward dementia. Research on vineyard workers in France indicates that these effects can reach measurable levels even in relatively young and healthy workers, particularly women.[128] In North America, researchers have discovered that youngsters with high levels of pesticide metabolites in their urine, particularly from foods grown with widely used insecticides like malathion, are more likely to have attention deficit hyperactivity disorder (ADHD).[129] After finding a doubling in ADHD rates associated with higher levels of petrochemicals in foods, the Canadian researcher who led this study recommended that parents shift their children's diets to organic foods.

FOR WHICH FOODS DOES ORGANIC MATTER MOST?

Knowing that pesticides and other chemicals can have negative health effects, consumers need to know which foods are the worst offenders.

Food News, from the Environmental Working Group, has a comprehensive list based on lab tests.[130] In general, thick-skinned plants like onions, avocados, and pineapples are the safest, whereas more porous plants like peaches, strawberries, and greens top the list of those for which it is most important to go organic. The list can seem counterintuitive in certain instances—thickness of the plant's skin is a key issue, but another significant factor is the extent to which heavy spraying or oil-based fertilizer use is commonly employed in growing a particular food.

CONCLUSION

Counseling on healthful dietary approaches is among the most important services provided by health practitioners. By providing evidence-based printed materials and through direct conversations with our patients, we have the opportunity to set an example for others to emulate.

Literature Cited

1. Mariman EC. Epigenetic manifestations in diet-related disorders. *J Nutrigenet Nutrigenomics.* 2008;1(5):232–239.
2. Doll R, Peto R. The causes of cancer: quantitative estimates of avoidable risks of cancer in the United States today. *J Natl Cancer Inst.* 1981;66(6):1191–1308.
3. Pomerleau J, Lock K, Knai C, et al. *Effectiveness of Interventions and Programmes Promoting Fruit and Vegetables Intake.* London, UK: World Health Organization; 2005.
4. U.S. Department of Health and Human Services. *The Surgeon General's Vision for a Healthy and Fit Nation.* Washington, DC: U.S. Department of Health and Human Services; 2010.
5. Slavin JL. Position of the American Dietetic Association: health implications of dietary fiber. *J Am Diet Assoc.* 2008;108(10):1716–1731.
6. Harvard School of Public Health. Health gains from whole grains. http://www.hsph.harvard.edu/nutritionsource/what-should-you-eat/health-gains-from-whole-grains. Accessed March 16, 2010.
7. Lichtenstein AH, Appel LJ, Brands M, et al. Diet and lifestyle recommendations revisions: a scientific statement from the American Heart Association Nutrition Committee. *Circulation.* 2006;114(1):82–96.

8. Bantle JP, Wylie-Rosett J, Albright AL, et al. Nutrition recommendations and interventions for diabetes: a position statement of the American Diabetes Association. *Diabetes Care.* 2008;31(suppl 1):S61–S78.

9. Kushi LH, Byers T, Doyle C, et al. American Cancer Society Guidelines on nutrition and physical activity for cancer prevention: reducing the risk of cancer with healthy food choices and physical activity. *CA Cancer J Clin.* 2006;56(5):254–281.

10. Doyle C, Kushi LH, Byers T, et al. Nutrition and physical activity during and after cancer treatment: an American Cancer Society guide for informed choices. *CA Cancer J Clin.* 2006;56(6):323–353.

11. Craig WJ, Mangels AR; American Dietetic Association. Position of the American Dietetic Association: vegetarian diets. *J Am Dietetic Assoc.* 2009;109(7):1266–1282.

12. Bischoff-Ferrari HA, Dawson-Hughes B, Baron JA, et al. Calcium intake and hip fracture risk in men and women: a meta-analysis of prospective cohort studies and randomized controlled trials. *Am J Clin Nutr.* 2007;86(6):1780–1790.

13. Lanou AJ, Berkow SE, Barnard ND. Calcium, dairy products, and bone health in children and young adults: a reevaluation of the evidence. *Pediatrics.* 2005;115(3):736–743.

14. Feskanich D, Willett WC, Stampfer MJ, et al. Milk, dietary calcium, and bone fractures in women:12-year prospective study. *Am J Public Health.* 1997;87(6):992–997.

15. Calcium re-examined: are you taking too much? *HEALTHbeat.*2008. http://www.health.harvard.edu/healthbeat/HEALTHbeat_052708.htm.

16. Jacobson MF. *Liquid Candy: how Soft Drinks are harming Americans' health.* Washington, DC: Center for Science in the Public Interest; 2005.

17. Physicians Committee for Responsible Medicine. Agriculture and health policies in conflict: how food subsidies tax our health. http://www.pcrm.org/health/agriculture/index.html. Accessed June 14, 2011.

18. Redwood D. Whole grains and beans as core components of a healthful diet: consensus, controversy and current research. *J Am Chiropractic Assoc.* 2010;47(3):18–26.

19. Mayo Clinic Staff. Whole grains: hearty options for a healthy diet. http://www.mayoclinic.com/health/whole-grains/NU00204. Accessed September 28, 2012.

20. Mercola J. http://www.drmercola.com. Accessed September 28, 2012.

21. Seaman DR. www.deflame.com. Accessed September 28, 2012.

22. Azadbakht L, Surkan PJ, Esmaillzadeh A, et al. The dietary approaches to stop hypertension eating plan affects C-Reactive protein, coagulation abnormalities, and hepatic function tests among Type 2 diabetic patients. *J Nutr.* 2011;141(6):1083–1088.

23. Uribarri J, Woodruff S, Goodman S, et al. Advanced glycation end products in foods and a practical guide to their reduction in the diet. *J Am Diet Association.* 2010;110(6):911–916. e912.

24. Tighe P, Duthie G, Vaughan N, et al. Effect of increased consumption of whole-grain foods on blood pressure and other cardiovascular risk markers in healthy middle-aged persons: a randomized controlled trial. *Am J Clin Nutr.* 2010;92(4):733–740.

25. Brownlee IA, Moore C, Chatfield M, et al. Markers of cardiovascular risk are not changed by increased whole-grain intake: the whole-heart study, a randomised, controlled dietary intervention. *Br J Nutr.* 2010;104(1):125–134.

26. Kennedy A, Martinez K, Chuang CC, et al. Saturated fatty acid-mediated inflammation and insulin resistance in adipose tissue: mechanisms of action and implications. *J Nutr.* 2009;139(1):1–4.

27. Johnston C. Functional foods as modifiers of cardiovascular disease. *Am J Lifestyle Med.* 2009;3(suppl 1):39S–43S.

28. O'Keefe JH, Gheewala NM, O'Keefe JO. Dietary strategies for improving post-prandial glucose, lipids, inflammation, and cardiovascular health. *J Am Coll of Cardiol.* 2008;51(3):249–255.

29. Nettleton JA, Schulze MB, Jiang R, et al. A priori-defined dietary patterns and markers of cardiovascular disease risk in the Multi-Ethnic Study of Atherosclerosis (MESA). *Am J Clin Nutr.* 2008;88(1):185–194.

30. Nettleton JA, Diez-Roux A, Jenny NS, et al. Dietary patterns, food groups, and telomere length in the Multi-Ethnic Study of Atherosclerosis (MESA). *Am J Clin Nutr.* 2008;88(5):1405–1412.

31. Giugliano D, Esposito K. Mediterranean diet and metabolic diseases. *Curr Opin Lipidol.* 2008;19(1):63–68.

32. Boldogh I, Aguilera-Aguirre L, Bacsi A, et al. Colostrinin decreases hypersensitivity and allergic responses to common allergens. *Int Arch Allergy Immunol.* 2008;146(4):298–306.

33. Anand P, Kunnumakkara AB, Sundaram C, et al. Cancer is a preventable disease that requires major lifestyle changes. *Pharm Res.* 2008;25(9):2097–2116.

34. Qi L, Hu FB. Dietary glycemic load, whole grains, and systemic inflammation

in diabetes: the epidemiological evidence. *Curr Opin Lipidol.* 2007;18(1):3–8.

35. Lutsey PL, Jacobs DR, Jr., Kori S, et al. Whole grain intake and its cross-sectional association with obesity, insulin resistance, inflammation, diabetes, and subclinical CVD: The MESA Study. *Br J Nutr.* 2007;98(2):397–405.

36. Jacobs DR, Jr., Andersen LF, Blomhoff R. Whole-grain consumption is associated with a reduced risk of noncardiovascular, noncancer death attributed to inflammatory diseases in the Iowa Women's Health Study. *Am J Clin Nutr.* 2007;85(6):1606–1614.

37. Esposito K, Ceriello A, Giugliano D. Diet and the metabolic syndrome. *Metab Syndr Relat Disorders.* 2007;5(4):291–296.

38. Esmaillzadeh A, Kimiagar M, Mehrabi Y, et al. Dietary patterns and markers of systemic inflammation among Iranian women. *J Nutr.* 2007;137(4):992–998.

39. Andersson A, Tengblad S, Karlström B, et al. Whole-grain foods do not affect insulin sensitivity or markers of lipid peroxidation and inflammation in healthy, moderately overweight subjects. *J Nutr.* 2007;137(6):1401–1407.

40. Qi L, van Dam RM, Liu S, et al. Whole-grain, bran, and cereal fiber intakes and markers of systemic inflammation in diabetic women. *Diabetes Care.* 2006;29(2):207–211.

41. Nettleton JA, Steffen LM, Mayer-Davis EJ, et al. Dietary patterns are associated with biochemical markers of inflammation and endothelial activation in the Multi-Ethnic Study of Atherosclerosis (MESA). *Am J Clin Nutr.* 2006;83(6):1369–1379.

42. Jensen MK, Koh-Banerjee P, Franz M, et al. Whole grains, bran, and germ in relation to homocysteine and markers of glycemic control, lipids, and inflammation 1. *Am J Clin Nutr.* 2006;83(2):275–283.

43. Giugliano D, Ceriello A, Esposito K. The effects of diet on inflammation: emphasis on the metabolic syndrome. *J Am Coll Cardiol.* 2006;48(4):677–685.

44. Mozaffarian D. Does alpha-linolenic acid intake reduce the risk of coronary heart disease? A review of the evidence. *Altern Ther Health Med.* 2005;11(3):24–30.

45. Lopez-Garcia E, Schulze MB, Fung TT, et al. Major dietary patterns are related to plasma concentrations of markers of inflammation and endothelial dysfunction. *Am J Clin Nutr.* 2004;80(4):1029–1035.

46. Esposito K, Marfella R, Ciotola M, et al. Effect of a mediterranean-style diet on endothelial dysfunction and markers of vascular inflammation in the metabolic syndrome: a randomized trial. *JAMA.* 2004;292(12):1440–1446.

47. Hauser R, Rice TM, Krishna Murthy GG, et al. The upper airway response to pollen is enhanced by exposure to combustion particulates: a pilot human experimental challenge study. *Environ Health Perspect.* 2003;111(4):472–477.

48. Jeerakathil TJ, Wolf PA. Prevention of strokes. *Curr Atheroscler Rep.* 2001;3(4):321–327.

49. Schulze MB, Hoffmann K, Manson JE, et al. Dietary pattern, inflammation, and incidence of type 2 diabetes in women. *Am J Clin Nutr.* 2005;82(3):675–684.

50. United States Department of Agriculture. *Dietary Guidelines for Americans, 2010.* Washington, DC: United States Department of Agriculture; 2010.

51. Guha N, Kwan ML, Quesenberry CP Jr., et al. Soy isoflavones and risk of cancer recurrence in a cohort of breast cancer survivors: the Life After Cancer Epidemiology Study. *Breast Cancer Res Treat.* 2009;118(2):395–405.

52. Thornton J. Is this the most dangerous food for men? *Men's Health*: *Rodale*; May 19, 2009.

53. Redwood D. The great soybean controversy II: misleading media narratives. *Health Insights Today.* 2009;2(6). http://www.healthinsightstoday.com/articles/v2i6/index.html. Accessed March 17, 2010.

54. Peeters PH, Keinan-Boker L, van der Schouw YT, et al. Phytoestrogens and breast cancer risk. Review of the epidemiological evidence. *Breast Cancer Res Treat.* 2003;77(2):171–183.

55. Petrakis NL, Barnes S, King EB, et al. Stimulatory influence of soy protein isolate on breast secretion in pre- and postmenopausal women. *Cancer Epidemiol Biomarkers Prev.* 1996;5(10):785–794.

56. Yan L, Spitznagel EL. Meta-analysis of soy food and risk of prostate cancer in men. *Int J Cancer.* 2005;117(4):667–669.

57. Krauss RM, Chait A, Stone NJ. Soy protein and serum lipids. *N Engl J Med.* 1995;333(25):1715–1716.

58. Erdman JW Jr. Control of serum lipids with soy protein. *N Engl J Med.* 1995;333(5):313–315.

59. Anderson JW, Johnstone BM, Cook-Newell ME. Meta-analysis of the effects of soy protein intake on serum lipids. *N Engl J Med.* 1995;333(5):276–282.

60. Sacks FM, Lichtenstein A, Van Horn L, et al. Soy protein, isoflavones, and cardiovascular health: a summary of a statement for

professionals from the American Heart Association nutrition committee. *Arterioscler Thromb Vasc Biol.* 2006;26(8):1689–1692.

61. Hegsted DM. Calcium and osteoporosis. *J Nutr.* 1986;116(11):2316–2319.

62. Warensjö E, Byberg L, Melhus H, et al. Dietary calcium intake and risk of fracture and osteoporosis: prospective longitudinal cohort study. *BMJ.* 2011;342:d1473.

63. United Nations University. *Protein and Amino Acid Requirements in Human Nutrition: report of a Joint FAO/WHO/UNU Expert Consultation.* Geneva, Switzerland: United Nations University; 2007.

64. U.S. Department of Health and Human Services, Food and Drug Administration, Center for Veterinary Medicine *The Judicious Use of Medically Important Antimicrobial Drugs in Food-Producing Animals.* Washington, DC: U.S. Department of Health and Human Services.

65. Hanrahan CE. *CRS Report for Congress: The European Union's Ban on Hormone-Treated Meat.* Washington, DC: Congressional Research Service; 2000.

66. U.S. Food and Drug Administration. *Report on the Food and Drug Administration's Review of the Safety of Recombinant Bovine Somatotropin.* Washington, DC : U.S. Food and Drug Administration, U.S. Department of Health and Human Services; 2009.

67. Chao A, Thun MJ, Connell CJ, et al. Meat consumption and risk of colorectal cancer. *JAMA.* 2005;293(2):172–182.

68. Micha R, Wallace SK, Mozaffarian D. Red and processed meat consumption and risk of incident coronary heart disease, stroke, and diabetes mellitus: a systematic review and meta-analysis. *Circulation.* 2010;121(21):2271–2283.

69. Larsson SC, Virtamo J, Wolk A. Red meat consumption and risk of stroke in Swedish men. *Am J Clin Nutr.* 2011;94(2):417–421.

70. Larsson SC, Virtamo J, Wolk A. Red meat consumption and risk of stroke in Swedish women. *Stroke.* 2011;42(2):324–329.

71. Larsson SC, Rafter J, Holmberg L, et al. Red meat consumption and risk of cancers of the proximal colon, distal colon and rectum: the Swedish Mammography Cohort. *Int J Cancer.* 2005;113(5):829–834.

72. Alexander DD, Weed DL, Cushing CA, et al. Meta-analysis of prospective studies of red meat consumption and colorectal cancer. *Eur J Cancer Prev.* 2011;20(4):293–307.

73. Alexander DD, Cushing CA. Red meat and colorectal cancer: a critical summary of prospective epidemiologic studies. *Obes Rev.* 2011;12(5):e472–e493.

74. Lam TK, Cross AJ, Consonni D, et al. Intakes of red meat, processed meat, and meat mutagens increase lung cancer risk. *Cancer Res.* 2009;69(3):932–939.

75. Cross AJ, Leitzmann MF, Gail MH, et al. A prospective study of red and processed meat intake in relation to cancer risk. *PLoS Med.* 2007;4(12):e325.

76. Cho E, Chen WY, Hunter DJ, et al. Red meat intake and risk of breast cancer among premenopausal women. *Arch Intern Med.* 2006;166(20):2253–2259.

77. Cross AJ, Freedman ND, Ren J, et al. Meat consumption and risk of esophageal and gastric cancer in a large prospective study. *Am J Gastroenterol.* 2011;106(3):432–442.

78. Tasevska N, Cross AJ, Dodd KW, et al. No effect of meat, meat cooking preferences, meat mutagens or heme iron on lung cancer risk in the prostate, lung, colorectal and ovarian cancer screening trial. *Int J Cancer.* 2011;128(2):402–411.

79. Tang D, Liu JJ, Rundle A, et al. Grilled meat consumption and PhIP–DNA adducts in prostate carcinogenesis. *Cancer Epidemiol Biomarkers Prev.* 2007;16(4):803–808.

80. Sinha R, Rothman N, Brown ED, et al. High concentrations of the carcinogen 2-amino-1-methyl-6-phenylimidazo-[4,5-b]pyridine (PhIP) occur in chicken but are dependent on the cooking method. *Cancer Res.* 1995;55(20):4516–4519.

81. Smith JS, Ameri F, Gadgil P. Effect of marinades on the formation of heterocyclic amines in grilled beef steaks. *J Food Sci.* 2008;73(6):T100–T105.

82. Gaby AR. *Nutritional Medicine.* Concord, NH: Fritz Perlberg Publishing; 2011.

83. U.S. Department of Health and Human Services, U.S. Environmental Health Agency. *What You Need to Know About Mercury in Fish and Shellfish.* Washington, DC: U.S. Department of Health and Human Services, U.S. Environmental Health Agency; 2004. http://www.mass.gov/eohhs/docs/dph/environmental/foodsafety/reporters04.pdf. Accessed September 28, 2012.

84. Debate Rages On Risk Of Mercury In Fish. CBS NEWS, August 19,2009. http://www.cbsnews.com/stories/2008/12/12/health/main4667226.shtml?source=RSSattr=Health_4667226. Accessed September 28, 2012.

85. Levi J, Segal LM, St. Laurent R, et al.*F as in Fat: How Obesity Threatens America's Future.* Washington, DC: Robert Wood Johnson Foundation; 2011.

86. Food and Agriculture Organization of the United Nations. *Livestock's Long Shadow: Environmental Issues and Options.* Rome, Italy: Food and Agriculture Organization of the United Nations; 2006.

87. Ornish D, Scherwitz LW, Doody RS, et al. Effects of stress management training and dietary changes in treating ischemic heart disease. *JAMA.* 1983;249(1):54–59.

88. Sacks FM, Ornish D, Rosner B, et al. Plasma lipoprotein levels in vegetarians. The effect of ingestion of fats from dairy products. *JAMA.* 1985;254(10):1337–1341.

89. Ornish SA, Zisook S, McAdams LA. Effects of transdermal clonidine treatment on withdrawal symptoms associated with smoking cessation. A randomized, controlled trial. *Arch Intern Med.* 1988;148(9):2027–2031.

90. Ornish D, Brown SE, Scherwitz LW, et al. Lifestyle changes and heart disease. *Lancet.* 1990;336(8717):741–742.

91. Ornish D, Brown SE, Scherwitz LW, et al. Can lifestyle changes reverse coronary heart disease? The Lifestyle Heart Trial. *Lancet.* 1990;336(8708):129–133.

92. Ornish D. Can life-style changes reverse coronary atherosclerosis? *Hosp Pract (Off Ed).* 1991;26(5):123–126, 129–132.

93. Ornish D. Reversing heart disease through diet, exercise, and stress management: an interview with Dean Ornish. Interview by Elaine R Monsen. *J Am Diet Assoc.* 1991;91(2):162–165.

94. Gould KL, Ornish D, Kirkeeide R, et al. Improved stenosis geometry by quantitative coronary arteriography after vigorous risk factor modification. *Am J Cardiol.* 1992;69(9):845–853.

95. Ornish D. What if Americans ate less fat? *JAMA.* 1992;267(3):362. author reply 363–364.

96. Ornish D. Can lifestyle changes reverse coronary heart disease? *World Rev Nutr Diet.* 1993;72:38–48.

97. Ornish D, Brown SE. Treatment of and screening for hyperlipidemia. *N Engl J Med.* 1993;329(15):1124–1125; author reply1127–1128.

98. Ornish D, Denke M. Dietary treatment of hyperlipidemia. *J Cardiovasc Risk.* 1994;1(4):283–286.

99. Gould KL, Ornish D, Scherwitz L, et al. Changes in myocardial perfusion abnormalities by positron emission tomography after long-term, intense risk factor modification. *JAMA.* 1995;274(11):894–901.

100. Ornish D. Serum lipids after a low-fat diet. *JAMA.* 1998;279(17):1345–1346.

101. Ornish D. Dietary fat and ischemic stroke. *JAMA.* 1998;279(15):1172; author reply 1172–1173.

102. Ornish D. Avoiding revascularization with lifestyle changes: The Multicenter Lifestyle Demonstration Project. *Am J Cardiol.* 1998; 82(10B):72T–76T.

103. Ornish D. Low-fat diets. *N Engl J Med.* 1998;338(2):127; author reply 128–129.

104. Ornish D, Scherwitz LW, Billings JH, et al. Intensive lifestyle changes for reversal of coronary heart disease. *JAMA.* 1998;280(23):2001–2007.

105. Ornish D. Very-low fat diets. *Circulation.* 1999;100(9):1013–1015.

106. Dunn-Emke S, Weidner G, Ornish D. Benefits of a low-fat plant-based diet. *Obes Res.* 2001;9(11):731.

107. Ornish D. Statins and the soul of medicine. *Am J Cardiol.* 2002;89(11):1286–1290.

108. Koertge J, Weidner G, Elliott-Eller M, et al. Improvement in medical risk factors and quality of life in women and men with coronary artery disease in the Multicenter Lifestyle Demonstration Project. *Am J Cardiol.* 2003;91(11):1316–1322.

109. Pischke CR, Weidner G, Elliott-Eller M, et al. Lifestyle changes and clinical profile in coronary heart disease patients with an ejection fraction of <or=40% or >40% in the Multicenter Lifestyle Demonstration Project. *Eur J Heart Fail.* 2007;9(9):928–934.

110. Dewell A, Weidner G, Sumner MD, et al. A very-low-fat vegan diet increases intake of protective dietary factors and decreases intake of pathogenic dietary factors. *J Am Diet Assoc.* 2008;108(2):347–356.

111. Frattaroli J, Weidner G, Merritt-Worden TA, et al. Angina pectoris and atherosclerotic risk factors in the multisite cardiac lifestyle intervention program. *Am J Cardiol.* 2008;101(7):911–918.

112. Govil SR, Weidner G, Merritt-Worden T, et al. Socioeconomic status and improvements in lifestyle, coronary risk factors, and quality of life: the Multisite Cardiac Lifestyle Intervention Program. *Am J Public Health.* 2009;99(7):1263–1270.

113. Dod HS, Bhardwaj R, Sajja V, et al. Effect of intensive lifestyle changes on endothelial function and on inflammatory markers of atherosclerosis. *Am J Cardiol.* 2010;105(3):362–367.

114. Nicholson AS, Sklar M, Barnard ND, et al. Toward improved management of NIDDM: a randomized, controlled, pilot intervention using a lowfat, vegetarian diet. *Prev Med.* 1999;29(2):87–91.

115. Jenkins DJ, Kendall CW, Marchie A, et al. Type 2 diabetes and the vegetarian diet. *Am J Clin Nutr.* 2003;78(suppl 3):610S–616S.

116. Barnard ND, Cohen J, Jenkins DJ, et al. A low-fat vegan diet improves glycemic control and cardiovascular risk factors in a randomized clinical trial in individuals with type 2 diabetes. *Diabetes Care.* 2006;29(8):1777–1783.

117. Turner-McGrievy GM, Barnard ND, Cohen J, et al. Changes in nutrient intake and dietary quality among participants with type 2 diabetes following a low-fat vegan diet or a conventional diabetes diet for 22 weeks. *J Am Diet Assoc.* 2008;108(10):1636–1645.

118. Barnard ND, Cohen J, Jenkins DJ, et al. A low-fat vegan diet and a conventional diabetes diet in the treatment of type 2 diabetes: a randomized, controlled, 74-wk clinical trial. *Am J Clin Nutr.* 2009;89(5):1588S–1596S.

119. Barnard ND, Gloede L, Cohen J, et al. A low-fat vegan diet elicits greater macronutrient changes, but is comparable in adherence and acceptability, compared with a more conventional diabetes diet among individuals with type 2 diabetes. *J Am Diet Assoc.* 2009;109(2):263–272.

120. Barnard ND, Katcher HI, Jenkins DJ, et al. Vegetarian and vegan diets in type 2 diabetes management. *Nutr Rev.* 2009;67(5):255–263.

121. Barnard ND, Noble EP, Ritchie T, et al. D2 dopamine receptor Taq1A polymorphism, body weight, and dietary intake in type 2 diabetes. *Nutrition.* 2009;25(1):58–65.

122. Levin SM, Ferdowsian HR, Hoover VJ, et al. A worksite programme significantly alters nutrient intakes. *Public Health Nutr.* 2010;13(10):1629–1635.

123. Trapp C, Barnard N, Katcher H. A plant-based diet for type 2 diabetes: scientific support and practical strategies. *Diabetes Educ.* 2010;36(1):33–48.

124. Redwood D. Are organic foods healthier? Health Insights Today. 2011;4(1). http://www.healthinsightstoday.com/articles/v4i1/organic-foods.html. Accessed September 28, 2012.

125. Dangour AD, Lock K, Hayter A, et al. Nutrition-related health effects of organic foods: a systematic review. *Am J Clin Nutr.* 2010;92(1):203–210.

126. Reganold JP, Andrews PK, Reeve JR, et al. Fruit and soil quality of organic and conventional strawberry agroecosystems. *PLoS One.* 2010;5(9):e12346.

127. Baxter GJ, Graham AB, Lawrence JR, et al. Salicylic acid in soups prepared from organically and non-organically grown vegetables. *Eur J Nutr.* 2001;40(6):289–292.

128. Baldi I, Gruber A, Rondeau V, et al. Neurobehavioral effects of long-term exposure to pesticides: results from the 4-year follow-up of the PHYTONER Study. *Occup Environ Med.* 2010;68(2):108–115.

129. Bouchard MF, Bellinger DC, Wright RO, et al. Attention-deficit/hyperactivity disorder and urinary metabolites of organophosphate pesticides. *Pediatrics.* 2010;125(6):e1270–e1277.

130. Environmental Working Group. EWG's shopper's guide to pesticides in produce 2012; 2012. http://www.ewg.org/foodnews/summary. Accessed September 28, 2012.

CHAPTER 10

Weight Management

Cheryl Hawk

THE OBESITY EPIDEMIC

Overweight and obesity were estimated to be the "actual" cause of 385,000 American deaths in 2000. This is only exceeded by tobacco use with 485,000 deaths.[1] In 2004, 17% of US children and adolescents and 66% of US adults were either overweight or obese. Of the 66% US adults, 34% were overweight and 32% obese. Furthermore, the prevalence of both overweight and obesity is on the rise.[2] The number of obese adults in the United States is currently 72 million, an increase of 2.4 million from 2007 to 2009.[3]

A body mass index (BMI) over 25 is associated with a greater risk for many chronic diseases. These include coronary heart disease (CHD), diabetes (type 2), hypertension, stroke, and cancer of the breast, colon, endometrium, gallbladder, and kidney. A BMI greater than 25 is associated with increased risk for less life-threatening but still important disorders such as gall bladder disease, musculoskeletal disorders, and sleep apnea. Obesity generally decreases the quality of life, because obese individuals have impaired mobility and are often subject to social stigmatization as well.[4] Children and teens who are overweight or obese have an increased risk for morbidity and premature mortality in adulthood.[5]

Overweight and obesity also impose a significant economic burden on the health care system. Overweight and obesity were estimated to be responsible for 9% of total medical expenditures of the US economy in 1998, and because their prevalence has grown from that time, this proportion may be expected to be even higher in the current scenario.[6] In the US, the total cost of medical care related to obesity was US$147 billion in 2008.[3]

ASSESSING OVERWEIGHT AND OBESITY

Several methods are in use to measure body fat, such as calculating BMI from height and weight, or measuring fat through bioelectrical impedance, dual-energy X-ray absorptiometry, or total body water. For the average patient who is not an athlete or bodybuilder, BMI is the most practical method for routine use in clinical practice.[7] BMI is calculated by dividing weight in kilograms by height in meters squared. BMI measurements are both highly reliable and valid, being strongly correlated with percentage of body fat.[8,9] Perhaps even more important, BMI has very strong external validity. This means that BMI in the overweight and obese category shows consistent and strong associations, established prospectively, to many negative health outcomes—as described above.[7,10] Furthermore, as BMI increases, the risk for negative health effects increases.[10] Therefore the U.S. Preventive Services Task Force (USPSTF) recommends screening patients in primary care for overweight/obesity using the BMI.[7]

BMI Calculation

There are many online calculators available to perform the BMI calculation almost instantaneously. The National Institutes of Health (NIH) provides one at www.nhlbisupport.com/bmi/ and also provides a table at www.nhlbi.nih.gov/guidelines/obesity/bmi_tbl.htm.

Figure 10.1 provides a summary chart for a quick assessment of BMI for adults. Table 10.1 summarizes BMI categories, along with associated health risks.

Text Box 10.1

DEFINITIONS

BMI: Body Mass Index

Overweight: BMI of 25–29.9

Obese: BMI of at least 30

Weight in Pounds			
Height	Normal	Overweight	Obese
5'0"	95-127	128-153	154+
5'1"	97-132	133-158	159+
5'2"	101-136	137-163	164+
5'3"	105-140	141-169	170+
5'4"	108-145	146-173	174+
5'5"	111-149	150-179	180+
5'6"	115-154	155-185	186+
5'7"	118-159	160-191	192+
5'8"	122-164	165-196	197+
5'9"	125-168	169-202	203+
5'10"	129-173	174-208	209+
5'11"	133-178	179-214	215+
6'0"	137-183	184-220	221+
6'1"	140-189	190-227	228+
6'2"	144-194	195-233	234+
6'3"	148-199	200-239	240+
6'4"	152-204	205-246	247+

Figure 10.1. Summary chart for determining BMI.

For children, BMI is calculated differently. The Centers for Disease Control and Prevention (CDC) provides a BMI calculator for children at: http://apps.nccd.cdc.gov/dnpabmi/Calculator. aspx

Growth charts may also be used to assess overweight and obesity in children. Overweight is indicated by placement in the 85th to 95th percentile in the growth chart, and obesity by the 95th percentile or higher.

In addition to BMI, it is important to assess central adiposity, since it is associated, independently of obesity, with increased risk of cardiovascular disease, diabetes, and other conditions. BMI does not measure the distribution of body fat, so it is important that both BMI and waist circumference (WC) be measured. The recommended method to assess central adiposity is by measuring WC.

Because almost all type 2 diabetic patients are overweight or obese, it is essential that the clinician be alert for the possible presence of diabetes or prediabetes, although the American Diabetes Association (ADA) recommends glucose screening only for those who have consistently elevated blood pressure. A 2007 study by investigators at the National Center for Chronic Disease Prevention and Health Promotion (NCCDPHP), CDC, found that the prevalence of adult-onset diabetes has almost doubled (from 5% to 9%) over the last 20 years. Obese people represented 81% of the additional cases, with over half of these having class II or III obesity (BMI > 35).[11] The ADA

TABLE 10.1	BMI and Waist Circumference Categories with Associated Health Risks			
	BMI	**Obesity Class**	**Disease^a Risk Relative to Normal Weight and Waist Circumference** Waist Circumference (in Inches)	
			♂ ≤ 40" ♀ ≤ 35"	♂ > 40" ♀ > 35"
Underweight	<18.5	—	—	—
Normal	18.5–24.9	—	—	—
Overweight	25–29.9	—	Increased	High
Obese Stage I (mild) Stage II (moderate) Stage III (morbid)	30–34.9 35–39.9 40+	I II III	High Very high Extremely high	Very high Very high Extremely high

Note: Increase in waist circumference can indicate increased risk even in those with normal weight.
^{a}Disease risk for type 2 diabetes, hypertension, and CVD.
Source: NHLBI Obesity Education Initiative. *Clinical Guidelines on the Identification, Evaluation, and Treatment of Overweight and Obesity in Adults: the Evidence Report.* Bethesda, MD: U.S. Department of Health and Human Services, Public Health Service, National Institutes of Health, National Heart, Lung, and Blood Institute; 1998.

SCREENING FOR DIABETES

Diabetes is defined as fasting plasma glucose of at least 126 mg/dL. The test should be repeated for verification on another day, especially if the first test results were close to normal. The American Diabetes Association recommends screening every 3 years.

Signs/symptoms suggestive of diabetes:

- Frequent thirst, urination, and hunger (polydipsia, polyuria, and polyphagia)
- Slow skin healing
- Frequent infections
- Vascular disease

Common screening tests:

- Fasting plasma glucose[a]
- 2-hour postload plasma glucose
- Hemoglobin A1c

[a]The American Diabetes Association recommends fasting plasma glucose; it is easy, quick, and low-cost, as well as convenient and acceptable to patients. It is also more reliable and less variable than, and has similar predictive value to, microvascular complications compared to the 2-hour post-load plasma glucose test.

recommends that anyone aged 45 years or older who is overweight should be tested for prediabetes, which is also referred to as Impaired Glucose Tolerance (IGT) or Impaired Fasting Glucose (IFG).[12] Younger adults should be tested if they are overweight and have additional risk factors such as hypertension, family history, or dyslipidemia. Text box 10.2 summarizes the assessment that should be considered for every patient with a BMI and/or WC above normal values.

Elevated lipid and cholesterol levels often accompany obesity and are one of a cluster of related modifiable risk factors of coronary heart disease (hypertension, diabetes, diet, obesity, and physical inactivity; tobacco is another important risk factor but is not closely related to obesity).[13] Total cholesterol and HDL–C screening for dyslipidemia should be considered for obese patients.[7,14] Table 10.2 indicates the categories for total cholesterol and HDL–C.

INTERVENTIONS FOR WEIGHT MANAGEMENT

Before describing a behavior-based, patient-centered, and individualized approach to weight management, we will describe several highly publicized approaches on which many patients may request information.

Weight Loss Drugs

Patients are often exposed to advertising or word-of-mouth discussions of weight loss drugs, so clinicians should be aware of the pros and cons of these medications. Two medications approved for long-term use, along with lifestyle changes, for obese people are sibutramine and orlistat. Although these drugs have produced modest sustained weight loss, continued use is required to sustain the weight loss. Sibutramine, which is a serotonin-norepinephrine- dopamine reuptake inhibitor, is structurally related to amphetamines. Thus, its side effects are like those of other sympatheticomimetic drugs: Dry mouth, increased blood pressure and heart rate, and so on. Any patient with cardiovascular risk factors should therefore be especially aware of such possible effects. Adverse effects of orlistat, which is a gastrointestinal lipase inhibitor, include fecal urgency, oily spotting, and flatulence.

Phentermine and mazindol are weight loss drugs only approved for short-term use. They

TABLE 10.2	Total Cholesterol and HDL-C Categories		
Risk Category	**Total Cholesterol**	**HDL-C**	**LDL**
High	240+	< 40	160+
Borderline high	200–239		130–159
Desirable	< 200	60+	< 129[a]

Note: Numbers represent mg/dL.
[a]This represents near optimal/optimal levels of LDL.

also have amphetamine-like effects, and adverse effects similar to those of amphetamines. Such side effects include dry mouth, dizziness, anxiety, insomnia, irritability, and constipation; more serious effects include rapid heart rate, chest pain, and difficult urination, and so forth. Furthermore, people rapidly build up a tolerance for these drugs.

Even though weight loss drugs are, in principle, supposed to be administered in conjunction with an appropriate diet and physical activity program, in practice, many people rely on the drugs. This of course results in only transient weight loss, and repeated cycles of "yo-yo" dieting.

The HCG Diet

The human chorionic gonadotropin (HCG) diet was first developed in the 1950s by Dr Albert Simeons. He theorized that HCG injections promoted fat burning, preferentially over muscle burning, on a very-low-calorie diet (approximately 500 cal per day), with little discomfort such as weakness or hunger and very substantial weight loss. However, later studies, including a 1995 meta-analysis of 24 studies, concluded that the evidence did not support these claims.[15] Even so, the HCG diet has been revived recently because the hormone is now available as a sublingual rather than requiring injections. The Food and Drug Administration (FDA) has not approved HCG for use as a weight loss drug. Furthermore, such low-calorie diets (<500 cal per day) do not provide adequate nutrients and may actually cause the body to shift into low metabolic gear. There have been some reports of adverse effects of HCG injections, including blood clots, headaches, depression, and dizziness, although the sublingual form has not been well studied. Women can also develop ovarian hyperstimulation syndrome (OHSS), which is a life-threatening condition. Symptoms of OHSS include severe pelvic pain, stomach pain, swelling of hands or legs, and shortness of breath. Perhaps most important is that the HCG diet does not foster changes in diet that can be sustained in the long-term and cause permanent weight loss, so any weight loss is liable to be temporary.[16]

Bariatric Surgery

Surgery is only recommended to be considered for people with a BMI greater than 40 kg per m^2 or with BMI $\geq$ 35 kg per m^2 and those who have not responded to other treatment, and who have severe health complications. It is recommended that a patient who desires bariatric surgery should be psychologically evaluated before being approved for the procedure. The most commonly used surgical approaches include gastric bypass and adjustable gastric banding. Bariatric surgery has produced large and sustained weight loss for extremely obese people. However, it has serious possible adverse events, the most serious of which is, of course, death, although the postoperative mortality rate is 0.2%. Other possible adverse events are wound infection, vitamin deficiencies, diarrhea, and hemorrhage. Furthermore, reoperation is necessary for up to 25% of patients who receive bariatric surgery. The long-term health effects of such procedures have not been thoroughly studied to date and have not been well defined.[7,10]

Weight Loss Diets—Do They Work?

In general, diet alone has not been shown to produce sustained weight loss.[17] However, patients are bombarded with advertising for special diets that will almost magically melt away unwanted fat within days or weeks. These "crash" diets that do not include medications generally fall into the categories of either *low-carbohydrate* or *very-low-calorie* diets. These are described below.

LOW CARBOHYDRATE DIETS

A 2008 systematic review of randomized controlled trials (RCTs) found that low-carbohydrate diets were more effective than low-fat or low-calorie diets in achieving weight loss and reducing cardiovascular disease risk at 6 months. At 1 year, the low-carbohydrate diets were still at least as effective, if not more so. However, the review suggested that more evidence, with longer follow-up, is needed.[18] There are many variations of low-carbohydrate diets. The 2008 systematic review only included studies restricting carbohydrates to a maximum of 60 g per day, although the studies actually identified were all based on restriction to less than 20 to 30 g per day at the beginning of the study, gradually increasing to as much as 50 g per day.[18] There was less attrition in the low-carbohydrate study groups than in the low-fat or low-calorie groups, even over 6 to 12 months, indicating that low-carbohydrate diets may be more acceptable. In most of the variations of low-carbohydrate diets, carbohydrates are gradually increased over time, to a maximum of about 100 g per day.

VERY-LOW-CALORIE DIETS

Very-low-calorie diets, or VLCDs, have been used for over 20 years to produce rapid muscle-sparing weight loss. They are considered modified fasts, with the maximum of 800 cal per day, often using a liquid protein supplement. They are recommended to be used only for obese individuals under medical supervision. It is important that individuals are carefully selected for this diet because of possible adverse effects, which include gallstones, muscle cramps, constipation, headache, fatigue, dizziness, electrolyte abnormalities, and hair loss.[19] In the 1970s, there were at least 60 US deaths from cardiac complications associated with unsupervised use of VLCDs, primarily due to liquid protein supplements made from hydrolyzed collagen that were inadequate in amino acids, vitamins, and minerals. These deaths occurred among people who stayed on the diet about 4 months; no deaths occurred in those who stayed on the diet only 2 months.

A 2006 meta-analysis found that VLCDs did not produce any greater sustained weight loss as compared to traditional low-calorie diets (providing 800 to 1,800 kcal per day).[19] Furthermore, traditional low-calorie diets do not require the same level of medical supervision as VLCDs and so are less expensive and more accessible to patients.

COUNSELING AND BEHAVIORAL INTERVENTIONS: A PATIENT-CENTERED, INDIVIDUALIZED APPROACH TO WEIGHT MANAGEMENT

"Counseling" means advising patients on how to change their behavior. "Behavioral interventions" is somewhat more structured, in that it refers to specific strategies through which people may learn skills, gain support, and become motivated to change their behavior related to weight management.

One of the simplest and most commonly used frameworks for helping patients change behavior is the 5 A's.[20,21] They are:

- *Ask* the patient about weight concerns ("How open are you to talking about weight management?"), diet, and physical activity—this information may also be collected on intake forms.
- *Advise* the patient on the necessary behavior change.
- *Assess* the patient's readiness to change, as well as risk factors present.
- *Assist* the patient in making the behavior and lifestyle changes, and following the action plan, including providing coaching/counseling, and information via fact sheets, pamphlets, and/or Websites.
- *Arrange* follow-up—this last "A" is essential, but is frequently neglected. Be sure the patients chart is flagged to ensure follow-up.

Research has shown that interventions that combine counseling on both diet and physical activity leads to greater loss of weight and abdominal fat than counseling only on diet, or physical activity. Furthermore, evidence also shows that high-intensity programs (contact with the patient more than once per month) and combining counseling with behavioral interventions are more effective, producing lasting weight reduction than moderate intensity (monthly contact) or low intensity programs (contact less than once per month). To achieve long-term results, follow-up is essential.[20]

As demonstrated by a large body of research, counseling by health care providers on health behavior related to both diet and physical activity can help patients achieve successful weight management.[4,7,17] The section below outlines an approach to such counseling. The KISS principle ("Keep it simple, stupid!") is important to keep in mind at all times, to foster sustainable lifestyle change. The CDC recommends some very simple steps to move toward a sustainable weight management program.

Helping the Patient Set Reasonable Weight Loss Goals

It is essential that the clinician assist the patient in setting reasonable, achievable goals for weight loss. The first step is to assess the patients

Text Box 10.3

SIMPLE SOLUTIONS

The Centers for Disease Control and Prevention recommend simple steps all Americans can take to combat obesity in themselves and their families.[3]

- Increase the number of servings of fruits and vegetables.
- Reduce intake of foods high in fat and/or sugar.
- Replace sugary drinks with water.
- Limit children's TV viewing to less than 2 hours per day—don't put a TV in kids' rooms.
- Breast feed babies.
- Support school, work, and community programs that promote healthy choices.
- Take a brisk 10-minute walk 3 times a day, 5 days a week (See http://www.cdc.gov/physicalactivity/everyone/guidelines/adults.html)

Please check the box that shows how ready you feel to start on a weight management program, where 0 would mean "not ready to start" and 10 would mean you've already started.

❏ 0   ❏ 1   ❏ 2   ❏ 3   ❏ 4   ❏ 5   ❏ 6   ❏ 7   ❏ 8   ❏ 9   ❏ 10

Interpreting the Readiness-to-Change Ruler
The following provides a general "rule of thumb" for assessing a patient's stage of change:
0–2: precontemplation
3–5: contemplation
6–9: contemplation/preparation
10: action

Figure 10.2. A "readiness-to-change" ruler for weight management.

readiness to make a change. Figure 10.2 shows a "readiness-to-change" ruler for weight management. Table 10.3 provides a checkbox format lassessment of the patient's readiness to start a weight management program. The clinician should be guided by the patients stage of readiness, as discussed in Chapters 2 and 3. Approaching the patient from the appropriate stage-of-change perspective will contribute to building his or her sense of self-efficacy. Self-efficacy develops with success, so achieving small, incremental goals contribute to it.

Dietary Component of a Weight Management Program
HOW MANY CALORIES?

A rule of thumb for determining a reasonable initial weight loss goal is 10% of the patient's current weight, within an interval of about 6 months.[4] For example, a patient who weighs 200 lb in January would therefore set a goal of reaching 180 lb in June.

For helping patients estimate the amount of calories they need to reduce, use another common thumb rule: One pound equals 3,500 cal; therefore, a reduction of 500 cal per day typically results in a weight loss of about 1 lb per week ($7 \times 500 = 3,500$). This is of course a very general rule, and many factors affect it, particularly physical activity, and the patient's individual metabolism. We will discuss this in more detail below; a combined approach in which caloric intake slightly decreases while caloric expenditure increases slightly is the best approach.

As described above, VLCDs have not been found to be more effective than traditional low-calorie diets, and must in any case be conducted with medical supervision among selected obese patients. Furthermore, "crash" diets do not help establish healthy, sustainable eating habits.

Most people will be amenable to, and capable of, cutting 300 to 500 cal out of their diet per day, if the clinician helps them identify the foods they would find easiest to cut. The best way to do this is to have the patient keep a 3-day food diary. Explain that its only purpose is to find out the most convenient place to cut 300 to 500 cal. Then, go over the diary and help the patient identify high-calorie, low-nutrient foods such as desserts, snacks, soft drinks, alcohol, and "hidden" sources of calories such as salad dressings, sandwich dressings, and sweeteners. Many people will find that all they need to do to cut 500 cal is to switch from sugary soft drinks to noncaloric drinks or, even better, water. Another easy cut is to switch to low-calorie salad dressing. Switching from fried to grilled meat; fruit as a side dish instead of french fries; and half a bagel with low-fat cream cheese instead of a whole bagel with regular cream cheese are all ways to significantly cut calories without feeling that one is making a huge sacrifice.

ENERGY DENSITY

Related to calorie reduction, research has shown that a successful weight management strategy is to replace high energy-density foods with those of lower energy density.[22] *Energy density* refers to the relationship of calories to weight of the food, measured in calories per gram. Table 10.4 gives examples of high, medium, and low energy-density foods. High energy-density foods have low moisture and/or high fat content. Most fruits and vegetables are low to very low energy-density, and so replacing higher energy-density foods with fruits and vegetables is helpful not only in terms of increasing fiber and nutrients, but also for weight management.

TABLE 10.3	Assessing a Patient's Readiness to Start a Weight Management Program
Statement	**Stage of Change**
❏ I'm not interested in doing anything about my weight right now.	Precontemplation—unwilling
❏ I'm not able to do anything about my weight right now.	Precontemplation—unable
❏ I'm thinking about doing something about my weight in the next 6 months.	Contemplation
❏ I'm planning to start a weight management program in the next month.	Preparation
❏ I'm in the process of starting an exercise program right now.	Action

FIBER

Another important factor in making sustainable dietary changes that will support a healthy weight is to choose high-fiber foods. Fiber is an indigestible portion of most plant-based foods, and not only helps with weight loss but also contributes to regulation of blood cholesterol levels. It is a preventive factor in certain cancers, and promotes healthy bowel function. It also provides a feeling of fullness, making it easier to maintain appropriate caloric intake. In fact, for some patients a more successful strategy than limiting calories may be to increase fiber, attempting to get at least 25 grams per day. This follows the principle discussed in Chapter 3, of accentuating positive actions and attitudes. Focusing on how to eat *more* foods with high fiber content is a more positive approach than focusing on how to eat less! It will help the patient to avoid feeling deprived. Food labels show fiber content, but easy ways of increasing fiber are:

- Animal products have ZERO fiber—fiber is found only in plant sources.
- Whole grains are good fiber sources; refined ("white") flour products are NOT.
- Legumes are good sources.
- Think: "**B**erries, **B**eans, and **B**ran."
- Foods advertised as "low carb" are often very high in fiber.

The Patient Must Take the Lead

The key factor in making successful dietary changes is that the *patient* decides which foods or beverages he or she can live without most easily, and which substitutions are preferable. "Being on a diet" is not a state one can perpetuate indefinitely; but cutting out a snack here and there, or eating a slightly smaller portion does not feel like "being on a diet" and is definitely sustainable. Understanding the importance of choosing low-calorie-density

and high-fiber foods is essential in allowing the patient to make informed choices.

Another useful principle in helping a patient devise a meal plan is that it is easier to take positive action than to stop oneself from doing something (which is a negative approach). Therefore, for patients who have gone through repeated cycles of dieting without a net weight loss, it may be helpful to use a form of positive reframing. Their goal should be to INCREASE fiber and vegetables, or to INCREASE water intake to eight cups per day, instead of REDUCING calories. Both of these goals can promote a feeling of fullness, although concentrating on what one is not allowed to eat tends to promote a feeling of emptiness and desire to consume more. Similarly, some patients may benefit by substituting exercise or deep breathing for snacking, especially during TV commercials, which are one of the most treacherous diet traps.

Physical Activity Component of a Weight Management Program

In terms of physical activity, it is also best to keep it simple: Any type of physical activity is better than none, and any duration, even if it's only 1 minute, is better than none. Patients who find it helpful to track progress can "rack up" exercise minutes without depriving themselves of TV shows they enjoy by using the commercial breaks to exercise, either with a pedometer, or simply by recording the minutes. Strength training exercises are readily incorporated into people's daily lives in this way as well. Chapter 7 covers physical activity counseling in greater detail. The next section addresses general approaches to help patients increase their physical activity.

HOW MUCH EXERCISE IS ENOUGH?

Increasing physical activity is a daunting prospect for most sedentary obese people. The CDC's current recommendation of at least 150 minutes of moderate activity per week—with added benefits from 300 minutes per week—can precipitate a feeling of hopelessness in many sedentary people. Thus it is important to start where your patient currently is, in terms of exercise. Also important is to help the patient identify ways to make exercise an integral part of everyday life. He or she should make a list of ways to increase physical activity seamlessly into regular activities, such as the following:

- Take a stretch break or short walk instead of a coffee break at work.
- Walk, step (with pedometer), stretch, or lift free weights during TV commercials.
- Use the stairs!
- Park further away from your destination in parking lots.
- Do it yourself!
- Wash your own car.
- Mow your own lawn; rake your own leaves; shovel your own walk; do your own gardening.
- Walk the dog—you'll both get more fit!
- Get your spouse and/or kids up and moving: Walk, play catch, and go to the park.

Two simple and easy approaches to increasing physical activity are *counting steps* and *counting minutes*.

COUNTING STEPS

Pedometers, or step counters, have been found to be successful in helping people increase their physical activity.[23–25] A widely used approach is to increase average steps by 2,000 per day; this is very roughly equal to 100 cal of energy expenditure per day. Figure 10.3 shows an "exercise prescription" and fitness calendar to use with a pedometer program. Many patients find the "instant gratification" of a pedometer very helpful, and can use their creativity to find ways to work extra minutes of activity into their daily lives: During TV commercials, parking further away from destinations, walking the dog, and so on.

COUNTING MINUTES

Counting minutes of physical activity does not require any equipment other than a watch. It is important that the patient identifies his or her current typical number of minutes of exercise per week, to allow for a gradual, and doable, increase of 60 minutes per week. This total can gradually be increased over time until it meets recommended amounts (150 minutes for general fitness, with 300 minutes conferring added benefits). However, at first, simply increasing it above their usual level will speed their weight loss. Sixty minutes of brisk walking, very roughly, burns about 500 cal, although of course this is highly dependent on current weight as well as many other factors. If 60 minutes is likely to sound too ambitious for a sedentary patient, rephrase this to indicate that 12 minutes of brisk walking—a much less daunting number—burns approximately 100 cal. Figure 10.3 gives a sample exercise prescription and fitness calendar for this approach.

Therapeutic Lifestyle Change

An intervention combining diet and exercise, and targeting dyslipidemia may be the best option for obese or overweight patients who also have elevated cholesterol. The program, Therapeutic Lifestyle Change (TLC), is recommended by the National Heart, Lung, and Blood Institute of the National Institutes of Health (NHLBI) for regulation of dyslipidemia.[26] The main components of TLC are:[26]

- Reduced dietary saturated fat (<7% of total caloric intake)
- Increased plant sterols (2 g per day) and soluble fiber (10 to 25 g per day) to lower LDL
- Weight reduction for overweight/obese patients
- Increased physical activity

TABLE 10.4	Energy Density of Various Foods	
High (4–9 cal/g)	**Medium (1.5–4 cal/g)**	**Low (0.7–1.5 cal/g)**
Cookies	Bagel	Fat-free cottage cheese
Bacon	Dried fruit	Most fresh fruits
Butter	Hard-boiled egg	Most vegetables
Crackers	Whole wheat bread	Skinless turkey breast

Name _____   Date _____

Exercise Prescription for Pedometer Program
- Measure your steps for 3 days. Divide total for 3 days by 3 to find your average steps.
- Increase your daily average by 2,000 steps per day
- Record your steps on "My Fitness Calendar" and bring on your next visit.
- Get help and information at www.AmericaOnTheMove.org

My Fitness Calendar

Exercise Goals   **Diet Goals**
Steps per day: _____   _____
_____   _____

Weight on Day 1 of Week 1: _____   **Weight on Day 7 of Week 4:** _____

Sunday	Monday	Tuesday	Wednesday	Thursday	Friday	Saturday	Week total
steps	steps	steps	steps	steps	steps	steps	steps
steps	steps	steps	steps	steps	steps	steps	steps
steps	steps	steps	steps	steps	steps	steps	steps
steps	steps	steps	steps	steps	steps	steps	steps
steps	steps	steps	steps	steps	steps	steps	steps

Name _____   Date _____

Exercise Prescription for Minutes Program
- Record how many minutes you exercise (walking, gardening, vacuuming) for 7 days.
- Add at least 60 minutes to your usual weekly total, for example, you could add:
- 10 minutes per day for 6 days OR
- 15 minutes per day for 4 days OR
- 20 minutes per day for 3 days
- Record your minutes on "My Fitness Calendar" and bring on your next visit.
- Get help and information at http://www.cdc.gov/healthyweight/physical_activity/index.html

My Fitness Calendar

Exercise Goals   **Diet Goals**
Minutes per day: _____   _____
_____   _____

Weight on Day 1 of Week 1: _____   **Weight on Day 7 of Week 4:** _____

Sunday	Monday	Tuesday	Wednesday	Thursday	Friday	Saturday	Week total
min	min	min	min	min	min	min	min
min	min	min	min	min	min	min	min
min	min	min	min	min	min	min	min
min	min	min	min	min	min	min	min
min	min	min	min	min	min	min	min

Figure 10.3. Exercise prescriptions for counting steps or minutes.

TABLE 10.5	Websites for Weight Management—Physical Activity and Diet
America on the move (pedometer program)	http://aom3.americaonthemove.org/
American College of Sports Medicine pre-exercise health assessment	http://www.myexerciseplan.com/assessment/
CDC basic nutrition information	http://www.cdc.gov/nutrition/everyone/index.html
CDC recommendations and tips on physical activity	http://cdc.gov/physicalactivity/everyone/guidelines/index.html
Fruit and veggies—more matters	http://www.cdc.gov/nutrition/every-one/fruitsvegetables/index.html
Let's move—Michelle Obama's program for increasing children's physical activity and improving nutrition	http://www.letsmove.gov/
President's challenge for increasing physical activity (join online groups)	www.presidentschallenge.org/
USDHHS program on healthy weight management	http://www.cdc.gov/healthyweight/losing_weight/index.html

Staying the Course: Follow-Up

The term "weight management" suggests that obesity should be considered a chronic condition, which requires ongoing attention. It is essential that patients who are overweight or obese focus on adopting long-term lifestyle changes which are not only acceptable, but actually enjoyable, if they are to be successful. This is why it is so important that they make small, incremental changes that they themselves identify as both important and achievable. The clinician not only assists in the initial adoption of these lifestyle changes, but also in following up to reinforce them. Another part of a successful weight management program is social support, as is indicated in the "wellness plan" structure introduced in Chapter 3 on wellness coaching. The office should maintain a file on programs and venues which patients can access to help them stay physically active and adopt healthy eating habits. Examples are YMCAs and fitness centers, health food stores—which often offer nutrition and cooking classes—senior centers, community centers, and churches. There are also many online programs (many of which also have local chapters for in-person meetings as well); examples of these are provided in Table 10.5.

To summarize, using the 5 A's mentioned at the beginning of this chapter to increase the effectiveness of any weight management program:

- *Ask* about the patient's willingness to discuss weight management, and about current diet and exercise habits.
- *Advise* the patient on what he or she needs to do to manage his or her weight successfully.
- *Assess* the patient's need and willingness to start the weight management program.
- *Assist* the patient in making lifestyle changes, including providing materials such as an exercise prescription and online or printed resources tailored to suit his or her needs.
- *Arrange* follow-up; flag the patient's chart to be sure you reinforce the program at each visit; link patients to community-based physical activity and nutrition programs.

Literature Cited

1. Mokdad AH, Marks JS, Stroup DF, et al. Actual causes of death in the United States, 2000. *JAMA.* 2004;291(10):1238–1245.
2. Ogden C, Carroll, MD. *Prevalence of Overweight, Obesity, and Extreme Obesity Among Adults: United States, Trends 1976–1980 Through 2007–2008.* Hyattsville, MD: National Center for Health Statistics; 2010.
3. Centers for Disease Control and Prevention. *Adult Obesity. Vital Signs.* Atlanta, GA: Centers for Disease Control and Prevention.; 2010.
4. NHLBI Obesity Education Initiative. *Clinical Guidelines on the Identification, Evaluation, and Treatment of Overweight and Obesity in Adults: the Evidence Report.* Bethesda, MD: U.S. Department of Health and Human Services, Public Health

Service, National Institutes of Health, National Heart, Lung, and Blood Institute; 1998.

5. Reilly JJ, Kelly J. Long-term impact of overweight and obesity in childhood and adolescence on morbidity and premature mortality in adulthood: systematic review. *Int J Obes (Lond)*. 2011;35(7):891–898.

6. Finkelstein EA, Fiebelkorn IC, Wang G. National medical spending attributable to overweight and obesity: how much, and who's paying? *Health Aff (Millwood)*. 2003;(Suppl Web Exclusives):W3219–226.

7. USPSTF. *Guide to Clinical Preventive Services*. Washington, DC: Agency for Healthcare Research and Quality (AHRQ); 2010-2011.

8. Gray DS, Fujioka K. Use of relative weight and Body Mass Index for the determination of adiposity. *J Clin Epidemiol*. 1991;44(6):545–550.

9. Deurenberg P, Weststrate JA, Seidell JC. Body mass index as a measure of body fatness: age- and sex-specific prediction formulas. *Br J Nutr*. 1991;65(2):105–114.

10. McTigue KM, Harris R, Hemphill B, et al. Screening and interventions for obesity in adults: summary of the evidence for the U.S. Preventive Services Task Force. *Ann Intern Med*. 2003;139(11):933–949.

11. Gregg EW, Cheng YJ, Narayan KM, et al. The relative contributions of different levels of overweight and obesity to the increased prevalence of diabetes in the United States: 1976–2004. *Prev Med*. 2007;45(5):348–352.

12. American Diabetes Association. Standards of medical care in diabetes–2007. *Diabetes Care*. 2007;30(Supp 1):S4–S41.

13. Helfand M, Carson S. *Screening for Lipid Disorders in Adults: Selective Update of 2001 US Preventive Services Task Force Review [Internet]*. Rockville, (MD): Agency for Healthcare Research and Quality (US); 2008. Report No: 08-05114-EF - 1

14. Pignone MP, Phillips CJ, Atkins D, et al. Screening and treating adults for lipid disorders. *Am J Prev Med*. 2001;20(Suppl 3):77–89.

15. Lijesen GK, Theeuwen I, Assendelft WJ, et al The effect of human chorionic gonadotropin (HCG) in the treatment of obesity by means of the Simeons therapy: a criteria-based meta-analysis. *Br J Clin Pharmacol*. 1995;40(3):237–243.

16. Robb-Nicholson C. By the way, doctor. I've been trying to lose weight for a long time and nothing seems to work. What do you know about the HCG diet? *Harv Womens Health Watch*. 2010;17(9):8.

17. Whitlock EP, Polen MR, Green CA, et al. Behavioral counseling interventions in primary care to reduce risky/harmful alcohol use by adults: a summary of the evidence for the U.S. Preventive Services Task Force. *Ann Intern Med*. 2004;140(7):557–568.

18. Hession M, Rolland C, Kulkarni U, et al. Systematic review of randomized controlled trials of low-carbohydrate vs. low-fat/low-calorie diets in the management of obesity and its comorbidities. *Obes Rev*. 2009;10(1):36–50.

19. Tsai AG, Wadden TA. The evolution of very-low-calorie diets: an update and meta-analysis. *Obesity (Silver Spring)*. 2006;14(8):1283–1293.

20. Whitlock EP, Orleans CT, Pender N, et al. Evaluating primary care behavioral counseling interventions: an evidence-based approach. *Am J Prev Med*. 2002;22(4):267–284.

21. Alexander SC, Cox ME, Boling Turer CL, et al. Do the five A's work when physicians counsel about weight loss? *Fam Med*. 2011;43(3):179–184.

22. National Center for Chronic Disease Prevention and Health Promotion Division of Nutrition and Physical Activity. Can eating fruits and vegetables help people to manage their weight? Atlanta, GA: Centers for Disease Control and Prevention; 2009.

23. Korkiakangas EE, Alahuhta MA, Husman PM, et al. Pedometer use among adults at high risk of type 2 diabetes, Finland, 2007–2008. *Prev Chronic Dis*. 2010;7(2):A37.

24. Murtagh EM, Murphy MH, Boone-Heinonen J. Walking: the first steps in cardiovascular disease prevention. *Curr Opin Cardiol*. 2010;25(5):490–496.

25. McNamara E, Hudson Z, Taylor SJ. Measuring activity levels of young people: the validity of pedometers. *Br Med Bull*. 2010;95:121–137.

26. National Heart Lung and Blood Institute. *Detection, Evaluation, and Treatment of High Blood Cholesterol in Adults (Adult Treatment Panel III)*. Bethesda, MD: National Institutes of Health; 2001.

CHAPTER 11

Injury Prevention*

Cheryl Hawk and Marion W Evans Jr.

PUBLIC HEALTH SIGNIFICANCE OF INJURY

Unintentional injury is the principal cause of death for Americans aged 1 to 44 years and is among the top 10 leading causes of death for all ages.[1] Tables 11.1 and 11.2 show the leading causes of death by age group, illustrating the prominent role of injuries. Both unintentional and intentional injuries (homicide and suicide) are among the chief causes of death in almost all age groups. Over 16% of the general population sought treatment for an injury in 2000, with resulting medical expenses of approximately US $117 billion. Injuries are also a significant cause of lost work time and both temporary and permanent disability.[1]

Is Counseling Patients on Injury Prevention Effective?

Most of the actions and policies comprising the field of injury prevention are implemented at the community level. However, health care practitioners can contribute by providing information, counseling on age-appropriate injury prevention actions, and increasing their patients' awareness of the importance of injury prevention to their health. They can also join in community activities supporting injury prevention, such as infant car seat and helmet use campaigns, and fall prevention and home safety interventions for the elderly.

Injury prevention and control is an area where a very large body of evidence has been developed, examining risk factors for injuries and evaluating methods to prevent them. The National Center for Injury Prevention and Control (NCIPC), part of the Centers for Disease Control and Prevention (CDC), was established with the mission of preventing injuries and violence, and reducing their consequences. The NCIPC addresses both intentional injuries (violence, including homicide and suicide) and unintentional injuries, the preferred term for "accident." *Accident* implies that the incident was unavoidable,

TABLE 11.1	Leading Causes of Death in US Children Aged 0 to 19 Years by Age Group				
Rank	<1 Year	1 to 4 Years	5 to 9 Years	10 to 14 Years	15 to 19 Years
1	Congenital anomalies	**Unintentional injury**	**Unintentional injury**	**Unintentional injury**	**Unintentional injury**
2	Prematurity	Congenital anomalies	Cancer	Cancer	**Homicide**
3	SIDS	**Homicide**	Congenital anomalies	**Homicide**	**Suicide**
4	Complications of pregnancy	Cancer	**Homicide**	**Suicide**	Cancer
5	**Unintentional injury**	Heart disease	Heart disease	Congenital anomalies	Heart disease

SIDS, sudden infant death syndrome.
Source: From National Center for Health Statistics, 2007 data, with permission.
Note: Intentional and unintentional injury causes are shown in bold.

* Portions of this chapter were adapted, with permission, from: Hawk C. Counseling on unintentional injury prevention: how chiropractors can help patients keep children safe. *J Clin Chiropr Pediatr.* 2009;10(2):671–675.

111

TABLE 11.2	Leading Causes of Death in US Adults by Age Group					
Rank	**20 to 24 Years**	**25 to 34 Years**	**35 to 44 Years**	**45 to 54 Years**	**55 to 64 Years**	**65+ Years**
1	**Unintentional injury**	**Unintentional injury**	**Unintentional injury**	Cancer	Cancer	Heart disease
2	**Homicide**	**Suicide**	Cancer	Heart disease	Heart disease	Cancer
3	**Suicide**	**Homicide**	Heart disease	**Unintentional injury**	COPD	Stroke
4	Cancer	Cancer	**Suicide**	Liver disease	**Unintentional injury**	COPD
5	Heart disease	Heart disease	HIV	**Suicide**	Diabetes	**Unintentional injury**

COPD, chronic obstructive pulmonary disease.
Source: From National Center for Health Statistics, 2007 data, with permission.
Note: Intentional and unintentional injury causes are shown in bold.

and most "accidents" actually have precipitating factors, which can be modified.[2] A general rule of injury prevention is that passive prevention—methods that act automatically and do not require people to remember to do something and take action—is far more effective than active prevention, where people must decide to voluntarily take a specific, appropriate action.[2] Airbags and childproof caps on medicines are examples of passive protection, whereas putting on one's seatbelt or supervising small children in the bath are examples of active prevention.

There are many proven methods to reduce risk factors for injury and to limit the consequences of injuries. These tend to be community based (e.g., soft surfaces in playgrounds) or legally mandated (such as the use of infant car seats and seat belts).

There are two areas of injury prevention where providers are most readily equipped to play an important role: Child safety and fall prevention in older adults.[3-5]

CHILD SAFETY

Child safety refers to safeguarding children from both unintentional and intentional injuries. Childhood injuries cause about 16,000 deaths annually in the United States; over 70% are unintentional and the rest are intentional. There are more than 20 million nonfatal injuries to children in the United States every year, with 300,000 hospital admissions and total costs amounting to US $347 billion.[3]

Evidence is building that health professionals, in clinical settings, can have a positive impact on

safety practices designed to correct some of the factors contributing to childhood unintentional injuries.[6,7] The evidence of the utility of health care providers counseling parents and children on injury prevention is such that in 1983, the American Academy of Pediatrics established The Injury Prevention Program (TIPP).[3] TIPP, which can be accessed at http://www.aap.org/family/tippmain. htm, includes comprehensive instructions for providers to ensure that they supply patients with the best injury prevention information.

Counseling is most effective when it is tailored to the child's developmental stage and to the family and social environment.[3] With infants or very young children, the parent and caregivers need to be the primary target for counseling, whereas older children should be included along with their parents in the conversation about safety. With adolescents, the primary target should be the teen, including the parents as support.

Specific topics that should be discussed with parents and children, by age group, are discussed in this chapter. Table 11.3, which lists the top three causes of fatal and nonfatal unintentional injuries, illustrates the issues that safety counseling should emphasize.[8]

Recommended Counseling on Child Safety, by Age Group

ALL CHILDREN

Health care providers should recommend that parents get training in cardiopulmonary resuscitation

TABLE 11.3	Leading Causes of Unintentional Fatal and Nonfatal Injuries Death in US Children Aged 0–19 by Age Group				
Rank	**<1 Year**	**1 to 4 Years**	**5 to 9 Years**	**10 to 14 Years**	**15 to 19 Years**
Fatal					
1	Suffocation	MVT[a]	MVT[a]	MVT[a]	MVT[a]
2	MVT[a]	Drowning	Drowning	Drowning	Drowning
3	Drowning	Fires/burns	Fires/burns	Other injuries	Poisoning
Nonfatal					
1	Falls	Falls	Falls	Falls	Struck/object[b]
2	Struck/object[b]	Struck/object[b]	Struck/object[b]	Struck/object[b]	Falls
3	Bites/stings	Bites/stings	Bites/stings	Overexertion	MVT[a]

[a]MVT, Motor vehicle transportation–related causes.
[b]Struck by or against object.
Source: From Centers for Disease Control and Prevention, 2000–2006 data, with permission.

(CPR) appropriate to their children's ages. They should also recommend parents that they post near the phone or program into their phone the numbers of local emergency medical services and poison control, and other emergency numbers.[3]

INFANTS

Most of the injuries to infants occur in the home or indoors, with the exception of motor vehicle (MV) injuries. The following topics should be priorities for families with infants:[3]

- Choking prevention: Parents should make sure children do not have access to objects large enough to lodge in their airway, or items like plastic bags and balloons. At a minimum, parents should:
  - Check toys for loose parts
  - Check curtain and window blind cords to be sure they are out of reach
  - Check all rooms and yard to remove small objects that could choke a child
- MV safety: Use infant car seats correctly— rear-facing in back seat; do not seat infants in the front seat with a passenger-side airbag. Small children should never be left alone in the car.[9,10] Parents need to wear their seat belts too! They not only serve as mentors to older

children to establish good safety habits, but seatbelted parents may reduce the risk of MV injuries for children as well.

- Water/bath safety: Infants most often drown in the bath or other containers; even buckets can be large enough to drown an infant. The best drowning prevention is to never leave a baby— even if he or she is in a bath seat—unattended near any body of water, no matter how small the body of water is.
- Fall prevention: Passive prevention devices such as window guards/locks and stairway gates are more effective than active prevention (such as picking the baby up when he or she gets near a hazard). For fall hazards such as changing tables, beds, and sofas for which passive prevention is impossible, infants should never be left alone even for a moment.
- Burn prevention: Parents should set hot water heaters to no higher than 120° F. All electrical outlets should be covered by childproof outlet plugs. Smoke alarms should be installed and checked regularly; one easy way to ensure this is to tell parents to check the batteries when the time changes in the spring and fall. Liquids should never be heated in the microwave because the heat is distributed unevenly and may burn the infant's mouth.
- Sleep environment safety: Soft materials or soft surfaces (feather beds, soft couch cushions,

pillows, etc.) are suffocation hazards. Always keep crib sides up and locked into place. Infants should sleep in a supine, rather than prone, position.

PRESCHOOLERS

Preschoolers should be introduced to basic safety rules so that these rules become habits. It is important to actively involve children in learning the importance of safety. However, this age group should not be relied on to implement all behaviors on their own. The following topics should be priorities for families with preschoolers:[3]

- Water safety: Preschoolers are less likely than infants to drown in the bath but more likely to drown in pools or spas. Such items should be safety fenced on all sides and have secure self-closing gates. Preschoolers should never be allowed to play in the water unsupervised.
- MV safety: Children over 1 year of age and weighing 20 pounds may sit in a forward-facing safety seat, although it is preferable to keep them rear-facing until they reach the highest allowable weight for the seat. They should always be placed in the back seat.[9,10] Preschoolers must be closely supervised around cars, including streets, driveways, and garages. This age group needs to start using helmets for tricycles and bicycles, even with training wheels.
- Fall prevention: Follow the same recommendations as for infants.
- Burn prevention: This is also the same as for infants, with the addition of keeping toddlers, who are highly mobile, away from oven doors, irons and iron cords, radiators, and heaters and grills. Parents should make sure hot liquids are out of children's reach.
- Poison prevention: In addition to keeping the local poison control number posted or programmed into parents' phones, all medicine, vitamins and other supplements, household cleaning and automotive products should be kept out of children's sight, preferably locked with childproof latches if possible. Ipecac, which had been considered a staple of poison prevention for many years, is no longer recommended. In fact, it is recommended that parents safely dispose of Ipecac they may have in the home.[11,12]
- Firearm safety: Firearms, especially handguns, should never be kept loaded; ammunition and unloaded guns should be kept in separate, locked cabinets.
- Prevention of other types of injuries: Sharp objects like knives and scissors should always be kept in a secure place; fans should always have childproof guards or should be kept well out of reach of children.

SCHOOL-AGE CHILDREN

School-age children should be actively involved in learning about safety and understanding the importance of their behavior. Parents also need to remember that they should model safety behavior with their children, such as always using their own seat belts in the car. Establishing good safety habits is extremely important. The following topics should be priorities for families with children in this age group:[3]

- MV safety: Children should graduate to a booster seat when they attain the highest allowable weight and height for their car safety seat. They should stay in the booster seat until they are tall enough to fit into the car's shoulder belt, which is usually about 4' 9".[9,10] Children should always wear helmets on bicycles, never ride in the back of a pickup truck, and should not use an all-terrain vehicle (ATV) until the age of 16 years.
- Water safety: Children should learn to swim at age 5, but should never swim alone. When boating, it is essential that they use approved flotation devices.
- Firearm safety: The same recommendations apply to children in this age group as to the younger ones. In addition, parents should ask their children if there are guns in any of the homes of friends they play with. Parents should instruct their children that if they ever happen to encounter a gun anywhere, they should not touch it and should immediately find and tell an adult about it.
- Sports safety: Each sport's safety rules, equipment, and conditioning should be observed and the adults supervising should make sure children adhere to them. Protective equipment for cycling, skating, and skate-boarding should be used.

ADOLESCENTS

Teens must be considered the primary target in discussions about safety, and it should be part of a discussion of healthy lifestyle in general. Parents should be considered their support system, while still respecting teens' desire for independence. Since peer pressure is very important in adolescence, schools and community groups need to be included as well, to diminish the opportunities for the risk-taking behavior so characteristic of adolescence. The following topics should be priorities for families with teens:[3]

- MV safety: Teens need to be engaged in discussions of the role of alcohol, drugs, speeding, and nonuse of seat belts in MV crashes. Discussing how to decrease distractions while driving is important. Parents should provide guidance and enforce rules limiting night driving and excessive numbers of passengers. Teens should use helmets when riding a bicycle, motorcycle, or ATV (although teens below age 16 should not drive ATVs).
- Water safety: Teens should be aware of the risks of swimming alone or in sites where swimming is not permitted, as well as of the risks of swimming or boating under the influence of alcohol or drugs. They need to be cautioned not to dive into any body of water unless they are sure of the depth and/or possible obstacles such as rocks. They should also use flotation devices during boating.
- Sports safety: The recommendations for school-age children also apply to teens.
- Firearm safety: The recommendations for school-aged children also apply to teens, and parents should recognize that firearms are even more dangerous to this age group because of their tendency toward impulsive action and risk-taking behavior, as well as the possibility of the presence of alcohol or drugs.

FALL PREVENTION IN OLDER ADULTS

Falls in older adults are an important public health issue, as well as an issue with which health care providers for older adults must be knowledgeable. Falls often result in decreased quality of life, disability, and/or death in older adults. Approximately one-third of adults aged 65 and older fall each year, and falls are the leading cause of injuries, as well as injury deaths, in this population. Of those fallers whose injuries require hospitalization, 40% to 50% subsequently lose their independence and enter a nursing home.[13] Related direct annual medical costs are at least US $19 billion, expected to reach US $44 billion by 2020.[14]

Assessment of Risk for Falls

The American Geriatric Society (AGS) clinical practice guidelines recommend that clinicians obtain a fall history from all older adults.[15] The Prevention of Falls Network Europe and Outcomes Consensus Group recommends defining "fall" as: "An unexpected event in which the participant comes to rest on the ground, floor, or lower level." They recommend incorporating this definition when taking a fall history, by asking patients, "Have you had any fall including a slip or trip in which you lost your balance and landed on the floor or ground or lower level?" The optimal interval for asking about falls has not been determined.[16,17]

Those who have experienced a fall should be screened for risk factors for falls. The most important modifiable risk factors are:[15]

- Impaired mental status
- Use of psychotropic medications, which may impair cognition and balance
- Polypharmacy
- Environmental hazards
- Poor vision
- Lower extremity weakness and/or dysfunction
- Impairments in balance, gait, and activities of daily living

Balance Assessment

There are a number of methods available to assess balance and gait. Two simple, yet valid and reliable, tests that do not require any specialized equipment are the One Leg Standing Test (OLST)[18,19] and the Timed-Up-And-Go (TUG) test.[20]

ONE-LEG-STANDING TEST (OLST)

The OLST requires only a stopwatch to perform. Instructions for the patient: With shoes off, stand on one leg, place your arms across your chest with your hands touching your shoulders. Do not let your legs touch each other. Look straight ahead with your eyes open. Repeat this procedure with the other leg.

The clinician times the patient until

- the legs touch each other;
- the feet move on the floor;
- the foot touches the floor; or
- the arms move from their start position.

Being able to stand less than 5 seconds on one leg is an indication that the patient may have a problem with balance.[21]

TIMED-UP-AND-GO TEST

The timed-up-and-go test (TUG) test requires a stopwatch, a chair, and masking tape to mark the floor. Instructions for the patient: Start seated in the chair. Stand up, walk 3 m (10 feet) to the mark on the floor as quickly and as safely as possible, cross the line marked on the floor, turn around, walk back, and sit down.

Patients who take more than 14 seconds to complete the test are likely to be at an increased risk for falls.[20]

Effective Interventions

The AGS recommends multifactorial interventions targeting specific identified risk factors. Interventions may include gait training, balance exercises, review and modification of medications, treatment of postural hypotension, hazard correction, and treatment of cardiovascular disorders.

- *Balance Exercises.* Balance exercises are recommended for recurrent fallers. Although optimal exercise parameters have not been definitively identified, the National Institute on Aging (NIA) of NIH recommends a set of exercises for older adults to improve balance and lower extremity strength.[22] These include the actions of plantar flexion, hip flexion, hip extension, knee flexion, side leg raise, single leg standing, heel-to-toe walking, and standing and sitting repetitions.
A 2010 systematic review funded by the Agency for Healthcare Research and Quality examined interventions designed to reduce falls in older adults.[4] The following interventions were assessed:
- *Physical therapy and exercise.* These interventions targeted (1) improvement of gait, balance, or functional training through exercises to improve strength, flexibility, and agility; (2) improvement of strength through resistance exercise; and (3) general exercise such as walking or other aerobic activity involving endurance.[4] For these interventions, the total contact hours (treatment intensity) ranged from 2 to 243 (median, 28 hours). In the pooled analysis, these interventions were found to reduce fall risk by 13% (confidence interval [CI], 6% to 19%). It was suggested that more intensive physical activity was associated with greater risk reduction.[4]
- *Vitamin D supplementation* reduced fall risk by 17% (CI, 11% to 23%) during 6 to 36 months

of follow-up. The evidence did not support an added benefit of calcium.[4]
- *Vision correction* was not found to decrease falls.
- *Counseling on fall prevention.* Counseling patients, without any other interventions, did not decrease fall risk.
- *Home hazard modification* was found to decrease fall risk by 7% to 41%, although overall only one trial found a statistically significant effect on fall risk.[4]

PUBLIC HEALTH SIGNIFICANCE OF MUSCULOSKELETAL INJURIES

According to the Bone and Joint Initiative (B&JI), musculoskeletal injuries or conditions are the most common causes of severe long-term pain and physical disability around the world.[23] In the United States, arthritis is the number one cause of disability and chronic spine conditions is number two.[24] Avoiding injury along with successful rehabilitation of these conditions is a major public health concern. Arthritis costs alone are expected to soar with baby boomers aging rapidly across America,[25] with the lifetime prevalence of arthritis around 80%.[26]

The B&JI estimates that 40% women over 50 years are expected to suffer at least one osteoporotic fracture in their lifetime[23] and many of these could be prevented with lifestyle changes and perhaps use of prophylactic medications. The B&JI scientists also estimated that traffic injuries would increase to the point that by the year 2010, they would be responsible for as much as 25% of all health care expenditures in developing nations and will result in many musculoskeletal injuries. In the US, conditions related to the musculoskeletal system cause more than 130 million patient visits to health care providers annually and are the chief reason people visit their physician, affecting nearly one in two Americans over the age of 18 years.[23] Back injury accounts for 27% of emergency room visits each year and 11% of hospital stays.[27] According to the National Institute for Occupational Safety and Health data released in 2000, there were 5.7 million work-related injuries and that about half of those injuries were to the back.[28] The report stated that over 60% were a result of overexertion, which would indicate these are preventable. In the report, males experienced two-thirds of the injuries and on average lost 6 days from work. There were also 119,000 traumatic, work-related bone fractures and half of those required 21 days off work. These injuries are often preventable and as one can assess, are very costly in both actual costs and costs in productivity. All clinicians should attempt to address any risk factor for unnecessary injury to the musculoskeletal system.

Literature Cited

1. CDC. CDC Injury Fact Book. Atlanta, GA: National Center for Injury Prevention and Control, Centers for Disease Control and Prevention; 2006.
2. Pless IB, Hagel BE. Injury prevention: a glossary of terms. *J Epidemiol Community Health.* 2005;59(3):182–185.
3. Gardner HG. Office-based counseling for unintentional injury prevention. *Pediatrics.* 2007;119(1):202–206.
4. Michael YL, Whitlock EP, Lin JS, et al. Primary care-relevant interventions to prevent falling in older adults: a systematic evidence review for the U.S. Preventive Services Task Force. *Ann Intern Med.* 2010;153(12):815–825.
5. Schnitzer PG. Prevention of unintentional childhood injuries. *Am Fam Physician.* 2006;74(11):1864–1869.
6. Kendrick D, Coupland C, Mulvaney C, et al. Home safety education and provision of safety equipment for injury prevention. *Cochrane Database Syst Rev.* 2007; (1):CD005014.
7. World Health Organization. *World Report on Child Injury Prevention.* Geneva, Switzerland: World Health Organization; 2008.
8. Borse N, Gilchrist J, Dellinger AM, Rudd RA, Ballesteros MF, Sleet DA. *CDC Childhood Injury Report: Patterns of Unintentional Injuries among 0–19 year Olds in the United States, 2000–2006.* Atlanta, GA: Centers for Disease Control and Prevention; 2008.
9. American Academy of Pediatrics. Car Safety Seats: a guide for Families. 2009. Washington, DC: American Academy of Pediatrics; 2009.
10. Biagioli F. Child safety seat counseling: three keys to safety. *Am Fam Physician.* 2005;72(3):473–478.
11. American Academy of Pediatrics Committee on Injury, Violence, and Poison Prevention. Poison treatment in the home. *Pediatrics.* 2003;112(5):1182–1185.
12. Bond GR. Home syrup of ipecac use does not reduce emergency department use or improve outcome. *Pediatrics.* 2003;112(5):1061–1064.
13. Lajoie Y, Gallagher SP. Predicting falls within the elderly community: comparison of postural sway, reaction time, the Berg balance scale and the Activities-specific Balance Confidence (ABC) scale for comparing fallers and non-fallers. *Arch Gerontol Geriatr.* 2004;38(1):11–26.
14. Whitlock EP, Orleans CT, Pender N, et al. Evaluating primary care behavioral counseling interventions: an evidence-based approach. *Am J Prev Med.* 2002;22(4):267–284.
15. American Geriatric Society. Guideline for the prevention of falls in older persons. American Geriatrics Society, British Geriatrics Society, and American Academy of Orthopaedic Surgeons Panel on Falls Prevention. *J Am Geriatr Soc.* 2001;49(5):664–672.
16. Hauer K, Lamb SE, Jorstad EC, et al. Systematic review of definitions and methods of measuring falls in randomised controlled fall prevention trials. *Age Ageing.* 2006;35(1):5–10.
17. Lamb SE, Jørstad-Stein EC, Hauer K, et al. Development of a common outcome data set for fall injury prevention trials: the Prevention of Falls Network Europe consensus. *J Am Geriatr Soc.* 2005;53(9):1618–1622.
18. Drusini AG, Eleazer GP, Caiazzo M, et al. One-leg standing balance and functional status in an elderly community-dwelling population in northeast Italy. *Aging Clin Exp Res.* 2002;14(1):42–46.
19. Maki BE, Cheng KC, Mansfield A, et al. Preventing falls in older adults: new interventions to promote more effective change-in-support balance reactions. *J Electromyogr Kinesiol.* 2008;18(2):243–254.
20. Shumway-Cook A, Brauer S, Woollacott M. Predicting the probability for falls in community-dwelling older adults using the Timed Up & Go Test. *Phys Ther.* 2000;80(9):896–903.
21. Maki BE. Gait changes in older adults: predictors of falls or indicators of fear. *J Am Geriatr Soc.* 1997;45(3):313–320.
22. National Institute on Aging. Exercise & physical activity: your everyday guide from the National Institute on Aging. 2004 www.nia.publications.org/exercisebook/ExerciseGuideComplete.pdf. Accessed December 1, 2012.
23. Bone and Joint Initiative. About the decade. http://www.usbjd.org/about/index.cfm Accessed August 31, 2011.
24. CDC. Prevalence and most common causes of disability among adults—United States, 2005.

MMWR 2009;58(16):421–426. http://www.cdc.gov/mmwr/preview/mmwrhtml/mm5816a2.htm. Accessed August 31, 2011.

25. United States Censsu Bureau. Press Release. Facts for features. Oldest baby boomers turn 60! http://www.census.govzuom.info/Press-Release/www/releascs/archives/facts_for_reatures_special_editions/006105.html. Accessed August 31, 2011.

26. Arden N, Nevitt MC. Osteoarthritis: epidemiology. *Best Pract Res Clin Rheumatol*. 2006; 20(1):3–25.

27. American Academy of Orthopedic Surgeons. The Burden of Musculoskeletal Diseases in the United States. Rosemont, IL: American Academy of Orthopedic Surgeons; 2008. http://www.boneandjointburden.org/about/index.htm. Accessed August 31, 2011.

28. Department of Health and Human Services. Centers for Disease Control and Prevention, National Institute for Occupational Safety and Health. *Worker Health Chartbook. 2000: Non-fatal injury*. No. 2002–2119. Cincinatti, OH:NIOSH Publication Dissemination; 2002.

CHAPTER 12

Tobacco and Substance Use

Cheryl Hawk

TOBACCO USE

Prevalence

As of 2010, the prevalence of cigarette smoking among US adults was 19.3%.[1] The prevalence was slightly higher in the Midwest (21.8%) and the South (21.0%). Of these smokers, 78.2% smoked every day. By state, smoking prevalence was lowest in Utah at 9.1% and highest in Kentucky at 24.8%. If current trends continue, by 2020, 17% of the US population will be smokers, implying that the *Healthy People 2020* objective of less than 12% will not be met.

Effect on Health

Tobacco use is the leading preventable cause of death and the actual cause of 18% of deaths in the United States.[2,3] This is more than the combined total from AIDS, alcohol, cocaine, heroin, homicide, suicide, motor vehicle crashes, and fires. The association between tobacco use and premature death is one of the best documented ones in the epidemiological literature, beginning with Doll's study of over 40,000 male physicians in 1951; this study then continued, following participants for 50 years.[4,5] Those studies showed that cigarette smokers had twice the death rate ratio as non-smokers (42% to 24%) for premature death (at ages 35 to 69 years). Cigarette smoking was found to be highly significantly correlated ($P < .0001$) with all causes of death, as was the number of cigarettes smoked, thus demonstrating a strong dose-response effect.[5] Table 12.1 lists some of the chief facts about tobacco use and its risks.[6]

Some studies suggest that tobacco use may be a risk factor for low back pain (LBP), and may contribute to poorer outcomes in people with musculoskeletal back pain, including outcomes of rehabilitation care.[7–9] A systematic review of smoking as a risk for LBP concluded that although the evidence suggests a link, prospective cohorts are needed to explore this link.[10]

Assessing Tobacco Use Status

The 2008 U.S. Department of Health and Human Services (USDHHS) clinical practice guideline on treating tobacco use and dependence recommends that all patients should be asked if they use tobacco, and clinicians should document this in their records.[11] It has been recommended that clinicians include tobacco use status in patient intake forms and clinic screening systems as a fifth vital sign.[11,12] The strength of evidence for this recommendation was designated as Level A, meaning that "multiple well-designed randomized clinical trials, directly relevant to the recommendation, yielded a consistent pattern of findings."[11] In a meta-analysis, it was found that just documenting patient report of tobacco use increases the rate of cessation interventions provided by clinicians (odds ratio [OR], 3.1; 95% confidence interval [CI], 2.2–4.2).[11] However, it also showed that use of a clinic system to identify and track patients' tobacco use status, alone, did not significantly increase rates of cessation (OR, 2.0; 95% CI, 0.8–4.8).[11]

Effective Interventions
COUNSELING

Community-based tobacco-control programs have been effective, judging by the decline in adult smoking prevalence in the United States from 29% in 1985 to 19% in 2003.[13] At the individual level, research shows that personalized physician advise influences patients to quit, when compared to patients not advised (OR, 1.3; 95% CI, 1.1–1.6).[11,14] Brief counseling (3 minutes or less) by a physician is effective in achieving long-term abstinence, compared to no intervention (OR, 1.3; 95% CI, 1.0–1.6).[11,15] Higher-intensity counseling sessions for more than 10 minutes achieve nearly twice the abstinence rates of brief counseling of less than 3 minutes (22.1% compared to 13.4%, respectively).[11,15] Use of state

119

TABLE 12.1	Tobacco Facts

Tobacco causes 400,000 deaths annually

US $150 Billion+ costs

US $150 Billion+ costs

About 21% of Americans currently smoke

50% tobacco users die from tobacco-related causes

Tobacco users die 10 years before nonusers on an average

Tobacco use increases risk of

     Lung and other cancers

     Cardiovascular disease

     Chronic Obstructive Pulmonary Disease

     Alzheimer's disease

The risks for smokeless tobacco are the same as tobacco smoking except for lung cancer; and it includes increased risk for mouth and throat cancer

Tobacco use risks are the same for men and women

Quitting significantly reduces many risks within a few years

Source: From U.S. Center for Disease Control and Prevention and Office of the Surgeon General, with permission.

Text Box 12.1

The 5 A's for helping patient quit using tobacco

- Ask: Identify tobacco use and record in chart
- Advise: Advise in clear, strong, and individualized terms that they should quit
- Assess: Determine stage of change with respect to willingness to quit
- Assist: Provide advice and resources (printed information and/or referrals)
- Arrange follow-up: Praise success and give positive support for those who relapse

TABLE 12.2	Tobacco Use Screener Assessing Readiness to Quit

Do you currently smoke or use other tobacco products?

❑ Never ❑ Formerly, not now ❑ Yes, currently

❑ I'm not interested in quitting right now.

❑ I'm not able to quit right now.

❑ I'm thinking about quitting in the next 6 mo.

❑ I'm planning to quit in the next month.

❑ I'm in the process of quitting right now.

❑ *Would you like to talk with the doctor about quitting?*

quit-lines for telephone counseling is also effective compared to no counseling or self-help only (OR, 1.6; 95% CI, 1.4–1.8).[11]

Step-by-Step Clinician's Guide: The 5 A's for Tobacco Users Willing to Quit

The use of the "5 A's"—*Ask, Advise, Assess, Assist,* and *Arrange*—is one of the most widely recognized approaches to tobacco cessation.[11] Text Box 12.1 summarizes the 5 A's.

ASK: IDENTIFY ALL TOBACCO USERS

Include a question on current and former tobacco use on the intake form (see Table 12.2). For current users, ask how long have they been using tobacco, what form of tobacco, and how much they use daily. For former users, ask how long ago they quit, how long they used it, in what form, and how much, to evaluate possible carryover health risks.

Alternatively, instead of asking tobacco use status as part of the patient-completed intake form, clinicians may prefer to include tobacco use status along with the patient's vital signs. This has been recommended by authorities on tobacco use cessation, since tobacco use status is as essential a part of the patient examination as the traditional vital signs.[12]

Be sure that every tobacco user's chart is flagged (such as by marking it with a colored label) to facilitate follow-up at subsequent visits.

ADVISE ALL USERS TO QUIT

Whether or not the patient is interested in quitting, it is important that the clinician make his or her position clear, from the perspective of a health care provider. However, it is essential that clinicians do not take a judgmental approach, as this is less effective than approaching the patient with understanding and empathy. A simple statement is all that is required at this point; it should be:

- Clear—"You need to quit smoking, and I can help you do it."
- Strong—"Quitting is the best thing you can do for your health."
- Personalized—use a "teachable moment"—relate tobacco use to the patient's current complaint, or his or her children's health (see Table 12.3 for risks related to secondhand smoke and tobacco use during pregnancy).[16]

TABLE 12.3	Health Effects of Secondhand Smoke

Children are at increased risk for:

Sudden infant death syndrome (SIDS)

Acute respiratory infections

Ear infections

Increased severity of asthma

Adults are at increased risk for:

Immediate adverse effects on cardiovascular function

Coronary heart disease (including heart attacks)

Lung cancer

Pregnant women and their babies:

Smoking by pregnant women causes 115,000 miscarriages and 5,600 infant deaths annually in the United States.

Pregnant smokers are at increased risk for:

Ectopic pregnancy

Placenta previa and placental abruption

Premature delivery

Infants of mothers who smoke are at increased risk for:

Low birth weight

Brain damage

Lung damage

Birth defects such as cleft palate or club foot

Babies of parents who smoke are at increased risk for:

Colic and fussiness

Poor sleep

Ear infection and respiratory infections

There is no risk-free threshold for exposure to secondhand smoke

Source: From U.S. Center for Disease Control and Prevention and Office of the Surgeon General, with permission.

ASSESS THE PATIENT'S STAGE OF CHANGE RELATED TO TOBACCO CESSATION

Ask every tobacco user if he or she is willing to make a quit attempt at this time. As shown in Table 12.2, this assessment may be incorporated into the intake form at the same time that information is collected on current and former tobacco use. The patient's stage of change will determine the best approach for assisting him or her. The stages of change, described in detail in Chapter 3, are:

- Precontemplation
- Contemplation
- Preparation
- Action
- Maintenance

Table 12.4 summarizes appropriate approaches for patients at each stage of change.

ASSIST—SUPPORT THE PATIENT IN QUITTING

The most important actions the clinician can take to support the patient's quit process are:

- Help him or her develop a quit plan
- Provide targeted counseling
- Provide a supportive environment with the entire office and staff
- Encourage the patient to identify and seek out social support
- Recommend and if necessary refer for supportive treatment, particularly tobacco-cessation medications
- Provide written information and resources to increase patient's self-efficacy.
- Each of these actions is described in detail below.

TABLE 12.4	Approaches to Assist Patients in Tobacco Cessation Based on Their Stage of Change	
Stage of Change	**How to Recognize Stage**	**Approach**
Precontemplation	No intention to quit in next 6 mo	Be nonjudgemental and show empathy
		Give personalized information
		Tell patient you are there to offer assistance when he or she is ready
Contemplation	Plans to quit in next 6 mo	Have patient list barriers and motivators
		Help patient develop strategies to overcome barriers
		Help identify support and resources
Preparation	Has already taken some action (such as cut down)	Encourage setting quit date
		Encourage preparing for quit date
		Get rid of reminders of smoking
		Rehearse strategies to deal with challenges
		Tell family/friends as ask for their support
Action	Has not smoked for 1 d–6 mo	Congratulate on success
		Ask if there are any triggers/problems; help identify strategies to avoid relapse
		Remind to reward him or herself regularly
Maintenance	Tobacco free for 6 mo+	Congratulate and support progress
		Continue to monitor health

Help Patient Develop a Quit Plan

First, he or she should set a quit date. Many people like to choose a day that has personal meaning, such as a birthday, anniversary of recovering from a tobacco-related health problem, July 4 (freedom from tobacco), the Great American Smokeout, and so on. Second, he or she should enlist social support by telling family, friends, and coworkers about it. Third, the clinician should assist him or her in identifying possible challenges and situations that may trigger a desire to use tobacco, and develop specific strategies to overcome each one. Fourth, he or she should get rid of tobacco and tobacco-related items to increase the difficulty of returning to the habit.

Provide Targeted Counseling

This does not mean that the clinician is functioning as a therapist; he or she is assisting the patient in exercising practical problem-solving skills and providing "moral support." Ask the patient about his or her prior experiences in quitting—"practice makes perfect"—to find out what worked and what didn't, to apply the successful strategies this time. Be sure the patient is aware of challenging situations and physical or psychological triggers and develop strategies for each one.

Counseling may be brief or intensive. Even brief counseling has been found to be effective. There is a strong dose-response relationship between frequency of counseling and effectiveness, so starting at the patient's first visit is important.

Provide a Supportive Environment with the Entire Office and Staff

Chapter 15 presents principles and details on retooling the office to emphasize wellness and health promotion in general. Large offices should appoint an office coordinator specifically for tobacco cessation, and all users' charts should be identified to be sure the staff and doctor provide verbal support at each visit. Posters on being tobacco free may be posted in the office, and brochures should be readily available in the waiting room. Buttons, pens, and magnets can be used to encourage patients to consider the issue of tobacco use, not only for themselves but for their family and friends. The Centers for Disease Control and Prevention (CDC) has many posters and brochures available at no cost (http://apps.nccd.cdc.gov/osh_pub_catalog/ PublicationList.aspx).

Encourage the Patient to Identify and Seek Out Social Support

It is especially difficult to quit if family members or close friends are still smoking. It is essential that the patient talks about quitting with his or her social network to be sure they will support, and not sabotage, his or her efforts. Some patients may want to attend a support group, especially if their family and friends are smokers. There are online support groups available, such as the WebMD smoking cessation community (http://exchanges .webmd.com/smoking-cessation-exchange).

Recommend and If Necessary Refer for Supportive Treatment, Particularly Tobacco-Cessation Medications

Quitting tobacco is very difficult, and medications have been found to be effective in assisting people to quit. Some are available by prescription and others are nonprescription drugs. Table 12.5 summarizes the medications most commonly used. Complementary and alternative medicine (CAM) therapies have less evidence, as yet, to support them, but since they are unlikely to cause harm, clinicians may want to suggest them to patients. Manual therapies, including chiropractic, osteopathic manipulation and/or massage, may help patients relax by decreasing muscle tension and helping to balance the nervous system, as they are working through withdrawal from nicotine. Both acupuncture and hypnotherapy have been used as part of a comprehensive approach to tobacco cessation, as well.[17] However, recent Cochrane

TABLE 12.5 Medications for Treating Tobacco Use and Dependence		
	Abstinence Rate % (95% CI)	**OR vs. Placebo (95% CI)**
Varenicline	33.2 (28.9–37.8)	3.1 (2.5–3.8)
Nicotine nasal spray	26.7 (21.5–32.7)	2.3 (1.7–3.0)
High-dose nicotine patch (>25 mg)	26.5 (21.3–32.5)	2.3 (1.7–3.0)
Long-term nicotine gum (>14 wk)	26.1 (19.7–33.6)	2.2 (1.5–3.2)
Nicotine inhaler	24.8 (19.1–31.6)	2.1 (1.5–2.9)
Bupropion SR	24.2 (22.2–26.4)	2.0 (1.8–2.2)
Nicotine patch (6–14 wk)	23.4 (21.3–25.8)	1.9 (1.7–2.2)
Long-term nicotine patch (>14 wk)	23.7 (21.0–26.6)	1.9 (1.7–2.3)
Nortriptyline	22.5 (16.8–29.4)	1.8 (1.3–2.6)
Nicotine gum (6–14 wk)	19.0 (16.5–21.9)	1.5 (1.2–1.7)

Source: From Fiore M, Jaen CR, Baker TB, et al. Treating tobacco use and dependence: 2008 update. Rockville, MD: U.S. Department of Health and Human Services, Public Health Service; 2008, with permission.

TABLE 12.6	Resources for Tobacco Cessation

"You can quit smoking—consumer guide"

U.S. Department of Health and Human Services, The Public Health Service. (June, 2000) http://www.askadviserefer.org/downloads/YouCanQuit_English.pdf

The new HHS Quit Line

800-QUIT-NOW

800-784-8669

Or www.smokefree.gov

"Making your workplace smoke-free: a decision-maker's guide"

U.S. Department of Health and Human Services, The U.S. Centers for Disease Control Office on Smoking and Health and The Wellness Council of America

http://www.fourcorners.ne.gov/documents/MakingYourWorkplaceSmokefree.pdf

TABLE 12.7	Health Problems Related to Binge Drinking

Alcohol poisoning

Fetal alcohol spectrum disorders

High blood pressure, stroke, and other cardiovascular diseases

Intentional injuries (firearms, sexual assault, and domestic violence)

Liver disease

Neurological damage

Poor control of diabetes

Sexual dysfunction

STIs

Unintended pregnancy

Unintentional injuries (MV, falls, burns, drowning)

STIs, sexually transmitted infections; MV, motor vehicle.

reviews did not find evidence that hypnotherapy or acupuncture is effective in tobacco cessation; more research is needed.[18,19]

Some authors have suggested that CAM practitioners are well-suited to delivering health promotion messages since patients see them as being supportive of prevention.[20] A survey of practitioners conducted in Arizona, Connecticut, Massachusetts, and Washington, found that CAM providers were more likely than mainstream physicians to record patients' tobacco use.[21] A feasibility study funded by the National Institutes of Health conducted in 20 private chiropractic practices with 210 patients developed a brief office-based intervention with promising results, suggesting that tobacco-cessation interventions are feasible in chiropractic practice.[22]

Provide Written Information and Resources to Increase Patient's Self-Efficacy

As stated above, the CDC has many posters and brochures available. Other resources are listed in Table 12.6. Clinicians should keep in mind that the written materials or websites recommended should be culturally, educationally, and age-appropriate for the individual patient.

ARRANGE FOLLOW-UP

To facilitate follow-up, it is essential to flag charts of all tobacco users. At the very least, ask patients who have quit or are preparing to quit how they're doing, at each visit. Be sure to praise and reinforce success, and assist with relapses in an empathic, nonjudgmental manner. Reframing the relapse as "practice" rather than "failure" is helpful—"practice makes perfect."

It is optimal to follow-up within 1 week of a patient's quit date, with a second follow-up within the month.

Tobacco Users Unwilling to Quit

For those who are not willing to quit, the "5 R's"—*Relevance, Risks, Rewards, Roadblocks,* and *Repetition*, is the recommended approach.[11]

RELEVANCE—EMPHASIZE THE PERSONAL RELEVANCE OF QUITTING

Relating the health effects of tobacco to the patient's chief complaint, or to his or her spouse and children may increase the patient's motivation.

RISKS—RELATE HEALTH RISKS TO THE INDIVIDUAL

Related to relevance, the risks of tobacco use need to be made real and relevant to the patient. For example, a young woman may not be motivated by the long-term risk of lung disease, but might be motivated to quit if she realizes that tobacco use prematurely ages the skin. What is sufficient motivation to one person may not be important to another. Parents may not be motivated by risks to their own health, but finding out that smoking negatively affects their children's health may be of much more concern to them.

REWARDS—IDENTIFY RELEVANT BENEFITS OF QUITTING

Again, rewards are valued differently by different individuals. Decreased risk of lung cancer might be especially important to a patient who lost a close relative to this disease, whereas improving respiratory function so that his snoring will not disturb his wife's sleep might be a key reward for another person.

ROADBLOCKS—IDENTIFY BARRIERS AND HELP THE PATIENT FIND STRATEGIES TO OVERCOME THEM

Once again, barriers are very individual issues. However, some of the most commonly experienced barriers are: Fear of weight gain, perceived inability to deal with stressful situations, and fear of failure in cessation.

REPETITION—MENTION TOBACCO USE AT EVERY ENCOUNTER

While always maintaining a nonjudgmental attitude, the clinician should continue to mention the issue of tobacco use at each encounter. It can particularly be helpful for patients who have made a number of quit attempts in the past for the clinician to encourage them to try again: "Practice makes perfect."[16]

Summary

See Text Box 12.2 for the U.S. Preventive Services Task Force (USPSTF) recommendations on tobacco use.[23]

- Tobacco use is the leading preventable cause of death in the US.
- Strong evidence supports the effectiveness of documenting patients' self-reports of tobacco status in their records in increasing clinician interventions for cessation.
- Brief counseling of 3 minutes or less by a physician contributes to patients succeeding in prolonged abstinence.

> **Text Box 12.2**
>
> U.S. Preventive Services Task Force Recommendations on Tobacco Use
>
> - *Grade A Recommendation:* Clinicians should ask all adults about tobacco use and provide tobacco-cessation interventions for those who use tobacco products
> - *Grade A Recommendation:* Clinicians should ask all pregnant women about tobacco use and provide augmented, pregnancy-tailored counseling for those who smoke
>
> Source: 2010 *Guide to Clinical Preventive Services*, U.S. Preventive Services Task Force.

- Counseling sessions for more than 10 minutes nearly double the abstinence rates of brief counseling (22.1% vs. 13.4%).
- Counseling combined with effective medication should be offered to patients without contraindications.

ALCOHOL AND OTHER SUBSTANCE USE

Effect on Health

ALCOHOL

Light to moderate alcohol consumption in middle-aged and older adults may provide some health benefits, including decreased risk for coronary heart disease. *Moderate drinking* is defined as less than or equal to one drink per day for women and people over age 65, and less than or equal to two drinks per day for men. Alcohol use is considered a health risk at the following levels:[23]

More than seven drinks per week or more than three drinks per occasion for women
More than 14 drinks per week or more than four drinks per occasion for men

Alcohol misuse is responsible for more than 100,000 deaths annually and is associated with both health and social problems. Men who consume an average of four or more drinks per day and women who average two or more drinks per day have significantly increased mortality, compared to nondrinkers. Heavy per-occasion alcohol use ("binge drinking") increases the risk of both injury and social/psychological problems, even when the person's average use is not above normal.[24]

SUBSTANCE USE (OF ILLEGAL DRUGS)

Marijuana and cocaine are the most commonly used illegal drugs in the United States; about 6% and 1% of the population, respectively, admit such use within the past month. Even smaller proportions of Americans use other illegal drugs, such as hallucinogens, inhalants, heroin, or methamphetamines. However, inappropriate (nonmedical) use of prescription drugs (analgesics, tranquilizers, stimulants, and sedatives), is increasing in the United States. Use of illicit drugs is one of the 10 leading preventable risk factors for years of healthy life lost, not only in the US but in all developed countries.[23]

Assessing Substance Use
ALCOHOL

The Alcohol Use Disorders Identification Test (AUDIT) is the most studied screening questionnaire. It is sensitive to detecting alcohol misuse and abuse or dependence. The four-item CAGE (feeling the need to **C**ut down, **A**nnoyed by criticism, feel **G**uilty about drinking, and need for an **E**ye-opener in the morning) is the most popular screening test for alcohol abuse or dependence.[23] A single-question screener developed and recommended by the National Institute on Alcohol Abuse and Alcoholism (NIAAA) has been validated for use in primary care to screen patients for unhealthy alcohol use:[25,26]

"How many times in the past year have you had *X* or more drinks in a day?" (*X* = 5 for men and 4 for women)

A positive response to this single-question screen is defined as any number greater than one.

SUBSTANCE USE

Although there are some valid and reliable standardized questionnaires to screen for drug abuse, their clinical utility has not been well studied. Clinicians should be alert to indications of possible substance abuse with patients, and follow up as appropriate. The current evidence does not support the concept of screening of the general population in primary care practice.[23]

Prescription Drug Abuse

Prescription drug abuse is a growing health problem in the United States. Although many prescription drugs can be abused, the most commonly abused drug classes are:

- Opioids, usually prescribed for pain
- Central nervous system depressants, usually prescribed for anxiety and sleep disorders
- Stimulants, prescribed for narcolepsy and attention deficit/hyperactivity disorder (ADHD)

Effective Interventions
ALCOHOL

Effective interventions to reduce alcohol misuse include an initial counseling session of about 15 minutes, with provision of feedback, advice, and goal-setting. Most interventions include follow-up. Multiple-contact interventions are more likely to be effective in reducing alcohol consumption, with effects lasting as much as 1 year after the intervention. These interventions may be provided in primary care by physicians or non-physician clinicians. However, it is recommended that providers receive training, or that trained practitioners and/or health educators, along with system supports such as reminders, prompts, counseling algorithms, and patient education materials, be used.[23]

SUBSTANCE USE

Evidence is insufficient to recommend interventions for substance use within the general primary care setting.[23]

Summary

See Text Box 12.3 for USPSTF recommendations on alcohol counseling.[23]

Text Box 12.3

U.S. Preventive Services Task Force Recommendations on Alcohol Use

- *Grade B Recommendation*: Clinicians should screen adult patients, including pregnant women, for alcohol misuse and provide/refer for appropriate behavioral counseling interventions to reduce misuse
- *Grade I Statement*: Current evidence is insufficient to assess the balance of benefits and harms of screening for illicit drug use

Source: 2010 *Guide to Clinical Preventive Services*, U.S. Preventive Services Task Force.

- Clinicians should routinely screen patients for alcohol use, and should follow-up with either referral or on-site counseling, if there are clinicians in the practice who have the appropriate training to provide an intervention.
- It is not recommended that clinicians routinely screen the general patient population for substance abuse, but should be alert to signs and symptoms of it in individual patients.

Literature Cited

1. U.S. Department of Health and Human Services. *The Health Consequences of Involuntary Exposure to Tobacco Smoke: A Report of the Surgeon General*. Atlanta, GA: U.S. Department of Health and Human Services, Centers for Disease Control and Prevention, Coordinating Center for Health Promotion, National Center for Chronic Disease Prevention and Health Promotion, Office on Smoking and Health, 2006.

2. Centers for Disease Control and Prevention (CDC). Smoking-attributable mortality, years of potential life lost, and productivity losses—United States, 2000–2004. *MMWR Morb Mortal Wkly Rep.* 2008;57(45):1226–1228.

3. Mokdad AH, Marks JS, Stroup DF, et al. Actual causes of death in the United States, 2000. *JAMA.* 2004;291(10):1238–1245.

4. Doll R, Hill AB. The mortality of doctors in relation to their smoking habits: a preliminary report. 1954. *BMJ.* 2004;328(7455):1529–1533. Discussion 1533.

5. Doll R, Peto R, Boreham J, et al. Mortality in relation to smoking: 50 years' observations on male British doctors. *BMJ.* 2004;328(7455):1519.

6. Centers for Disease Control and Prevention (CDC). Tobacco use among adults—United States, 2005. *MMWR Morb Mortal Wkly Rep.* 2006;55(42):1145–1148.

7. Pincus T, Santos R, Breen A, et al. A review and proposal for a core set of factors for prospective cohorts in low back pain: a consensus statement. *Arthritis Rheum.* 2008;59(1).14–24.

8. Rushtine GR II, Crawley W, Castellvi A, et al. Effect of the spine practitioner on patient smoking status. *Spine (Phila Pa 1976).* 2000;25(17):2229–2233.

9. McGeary DD, Mayer TG, Gatchel RJ, et al. Smoking status and psychosocioeconomic outcomes of functional restoration in patients with chronic spinal disability. *Spine J.* 2004;4(2):170–175.

10. Goldberg MS, Scott SC, Mayo NE. A review of the association between cigarette smoking and the development of nonspecific back pain and related outcomes. *Spine (Phila Pa 1976).* 2000;25(8):995–1014.

11. Fiore M, Jaén CR, Baker TB, et al. Treating tobacco use and dependence: 2008 update. Rockville, MD: U.S. Department of Health and Human Services, Public Health Service; 2008.

12. Ahluwalia JS, Gibson CA, Kenney RE, et al. Smoking status as a vital sign. *J Gen Intern Med.* 1999;14(7):402–408.

13. Farelley MC, Pechacek TF, Thomas KY, et al. The impact of tobacco control programs on adult smoking. *Am J Public Health.* 2008;98(2):304–309.

14. Kreuter MW, Chheda SG, Bull FC. How does physician advice influence patient behavior? Evidence for a priming effect. *Arch Fam Med.* 2000;9(5):426–433.

15. Hays JT, Ebbert JO, Sood A. Treating tobacco dependence in light of the 2008 US Department of Health and Human Services clinical practice guideline. *Mayo Clin Proc.* 2009;84(8):730–735; quiz 735–736.

16. U.S. Surgeon General. *Health Consequences of Involuntary Exposure to Tobacco Smoke*. Rockville, MD: U.S. Department of Health and Human Services; 2007.

17. Evans M, Leach RA, Cohen IA, et al. A multidisciplinary approach to counseling a 65-year-old woman on smoking cessation. *Topics in Integrative Health Care.* 2010;1(1).

18. Barnes J, Dong CY, McRobbie H, et al. Hypnotherapy for smoking cessation. *Cochrane Database Syst Rev.* 2010;(10):CD001008.

19. White AR, Rampes H, Liu JP, et al. Acupuncture and related interventions for smoking cessation. *Cochrane Database Syst Rev.* 2011;(1):CD000009.

20. Hill FJ. Complementary and alternative medicine: the next generation of health promotion? *Health Promot Int.* 2003;18(3):265–272.

21. Cherkin DC, Deyo RA, Sherman KJ, et al. Characteristics of visits to licensed acupuncturists, chiropractors, massage therapists, and naturopathic physicians. *J Am Board Fam Pract.* 2002;15(6):463–472.

22. Gordon JS, Istvan J, Haas M. Tobacco cessation via doctors of chiropractic: results of a feasibility study. *Nicotine Tob Res.* 2010;12(3):305–308.

23. USPSTF. *Guide to Clinical Preventive Services.* Washington, DC: Agency for Healthcare Research and Quality (AHRQ); 2010.

24. Whitlock EP, Polen MR, Green CA, et al. Behavioral counseling interventions in primary care to reduce risky/harmful alcohol use by adults: a summary of the evidence for the U.S. Preventive Services Task Force. *Ann Intern Med.* 2004;140(7):557–568.

25. Smith PC, Schmidt SM, Allensworth-Davies D, et al. Primary care validation of a single-question alcohol screening test. *J Gen Intern Med.* 2009;24(7):783–788.

26. National Institute on Alcohol Abuse and Alcoholism. *Helping Patients Who Drink too Much: a Clinician's Guide.* Bethesda, MD: NIAAA; 2007.

CHAPTER 13

Stress Management and Stress-Related Conditions

Cheryl Hawk

OVERVIEW OF STRESS

Stress is an unavoidable part of modern life. An American Psychological Association survey carried out in 2007 found that 75% of Americans report experiencing symptoms of stress in the past month; 48% say that their stress has increased within the past 5 years.[1] Stress is implicated in a growing number of chronic conditions, including hypertension, metabolic syndrome, cardiovascular disease, mental disorders, and musculoskeletal dysfunction.[2–5] However, the term "stress" should actually be modified to indicate that the actual culprit in contributing to chronic disease is a person's reaction to stress, rather than the stressor or amount of stress present in the environment. That is, it is *distress*, not simply *stress*, which is the problem. Stress itself is neither positive nor negative; it is, according to Selye's classic definition, simply "the non-specific response of the body to any demand placed upon it."[6] The body is designed to accommodate stress through the action of the sympathetic nervous system (SNS). These actions are to:

- Increase heart rate
- Increase blood pressure
- Increase blood sugar level
- Increase respiration rate
- Increase muscle tension
- Increase rate of blood clotting
- Decrease digestive process

This physiology of the stress reaction becomes more complex when it becomes a chronic state in which the individual is constantly "on red alert." Multiple bodily systems become involved as the body attempts to handle a chronic imbalance in which the SNS, which is designed to handle emergencies only, is overactive. The immune system, mental and psychological state, appetite, sexual function are all affected by this state of imbalance, leading to a host of symptoms

and functional and even, eventually, structural disorders.

Stress is often categorized by the type of situation that evokes—in a susceptible individual—a stress reaction. These are (1) harm or loss (e.g., death of a loved one, being attacked or robbed, being injured in a car crash, etc.); (2) threats (i.e., feeling "up against it" in everyday life; e.g., being chastised by a superior at work, failing a course in school, getting a traffic ticket, etc.); and (3) challenges (i.e., experiencing a life change; e.g., moving to a new location, graduating from college, getting married, etc.).[7]

Obviously, different people will experience widely different situations as being stressful. The core issue in management of chronic stress is *control*. People who react with a prolonged and continuing "fight or flight" response to ordinary situations tend to feel a lack of control, so that almost any occurrence can feel like a possible loss, threat, or challenge. Thus, the central principle of stress management is to empower the patient with a sense of control—that is, self-efficacy. This concept was discussed in detail in Chapter 2. In this chapter, we will consider methods that will increase the patient's feeling of self-efficacy with respect to stressful situations in his or her life.

ASSESSMENT OF STRESS

There are a number of questionnaires in use to assess an individual's stress level. They can be categorized as those which evaluate external stress—that is, life events perceived as stressful—and those which evaluate the individual's internal reaction to stress. In terms of assisting patients to achieve self-efficacy in stress management, it is most useful to help them evaluate their reaction to stress, rather than computing how high their external stress levels are. That is, we can't control outside events which cause stress, but we can control our reaction to these events—the term "stress management" refers more to managing our reaction than to managing the occurrence of stressful events. Learning to control our reaction to stress provides a feeling of control and empowerment.

Numeric Rating Scales

The simplest way to evaluate stress is to use a numeric rating scale (NRS). This is often done by asking, "On a scale of 0 to 10, where 0 is no stress and 10 is unbearable stress, how would you rate your current stress level?"

However, in keeping with the coaching principle that it is important to frame concepts in a positive manner, and in a way that encourages self-efficacy, it is usually more helpful to emphasize the person's ability to manage whatever stress he is experiencing, rather than focusing on the perceived degree of stress present. That is

> "On a scale of 0 to 10, where 0 is no confidence and 10 is complete confidence, how confident are you that you can successfully manage your current stress level? That is, manage it without negatively affecting your health and well-being?"

This approach evaluates the patient's *confidence* rather than her external influences, which is the appropriate perspective for beginning counseling in stress management.

Some instruments commonly used in psychology, such as the Perceived Stress Scale, also tend to focus on the individuals rather than life events, asking about their confidence in their ability to handle stress, and to control important things in life.[8] However, other popular instruments such as Holmes and Rahe Social Readjustment Rating Scale focus instead on scoring the degree of stress, usually in terms of events, currently present in the individual's life, to assess his or her likelihood of suffering stress-related illness.[9] Although this may be helpful in showing the patient the importance of learning stress management skills by providing a teachable moment, it tends to shift the locus of control away from the individual.

STRESS MANAGEMENT

It is important to keep in mind the concept of self-efficacy when assisting a patient in developing an approach to managing stress. Stress management is not a one-size-fits-all activity. Although evidence-based approaches are preferable, the most important factor is the "fit" of the approach to the patient's preferences, values, and abilities.[10]

A patient who is very much oriented toward conventional thinking and materialism may not find meditation to be to his taste, whereas one who dislikes exercise and has chronic pain may not be immediately open to tai chi. Both meditation and tai chi are known to help in stress management and improving quality of life,[11,12] but if the patient is unwilling, they will be useless.

Thus it is important to begin stress management with a common denominator factor to which almost any patient can relate, and which is closely tied to stress reactions: Sleep quality.

The Role of Sleep Quality in Stress Management

Poor sleep can be caused by stress and also contributes to stress. This is a continuing feedback loop, which must be curtailed. Nearly half (40%) of US adults get fewer than 7 hours of sleep each night, and the same proportion either cannot fall asleep easily at night or become drowsy during the day—or both. Insomnia is diagnosed chiefly by the patient reporting difficulty with falling asleep or staying asleep. Insomnia is closely related to stress reactions in that it is considered to be associated with a state of hyperarousal, which, of course suggests involvement of the SNS. Some studies have found that both cortisol and adrenocorticotropic hormone (ACTH) levels are elevated in people with insomnia, compared to those without sleep complaints, suggesting activation of the hypothalamic–pituitary–adrenal (HPA) axis.[13,14] Although this appears to be a "which came first, the chicken or the egg?" situation, improving one's sleep quality can make an important contribution to successful stress management. Insomnia, alone, is known to contribute directly to a lower quality of life, impaired function in everyday life, and it also increases the risk of depression and anxiety. It may also contribute to cardiovascular disease, and obesity and metabolic syndrome.[13,15]

It is estimated that annually, about 25% of Americans take some type of sleep medication. Neither prescription nor nonprescription medications are without side effects; these are summarized in Table 13.1. Herbal and other nonprescription supplements are less likely to cause side effects or dependence, but less is known about their effectiveness. Although the research is not definitive, melatonin and valerian root supplements appear to have benefits and their side effects are low.[16–18] In fact, melatonin has been used successfully to replace hypnotics in older adults.[19]

TABLE 13.1	Prescription and Nonprescription Medications for Insomnia		
Drug Class	**Examples of Generic/ Brand Names**	**Side Effects**	**Potential for Dependence and Abuse**
Prescription			
Benzodiazepine hypnotics	Flurazepam (Dalmane), Clonazepam (Klonopin); Triazolam (Halcion), Lorazepam (Ativan), Alprazolam (Xanax), Temazepam (Restoril), Oxazepam (Serax), Flunitrazepam (Rohypnol)	Worsening of depression; daytime drowsiness increasing risk of accidents and falls; memory loss; urinary incontinence; performing activities while asleep (driving, cooking, and binge eating)	High
Nonbenzodiazepine hypnotics	Zolpidem (Ambien) Zaleplon (Sonata) Eszopiclone (Lunesta) Ramelteon (Rozerem)	Less pronounced than benzodiazepines; morning drowsiness, memory loss, performing activities while asleep (driving, cooking, and binge eating)	Less than benzodiazepines; ramelteon the least
Antidepressants	Trazodone, doxepin, trimipramine, amitriptyline, and mirtazipine.	Daytime drowsiness, dizziness	Low
Nonprescription Medications			
Antihistamines	Diphenhydramine (Benadryl, Nytol, Sleep-Eez, Sominex) Doxylamine (Unison)	Daytime drowsiness, cognitive impairment, dizziness, blurred vision, clumsiness, and dry mouth	Low

The same interventions that help with stress management also address insomnia. However, there are also factors that are specific for insomnia. One of the most important factors is avoiding caffeine. Most patients do not realize that caffeine can stay in their system for as long as 10 hours, so, as a general rule, it is important to restrict caffeinated beverages (coffee, tea, cola, and energy drinks) to mornings. It is recommended that total caffeine consumption should be less than 300 mg per day (one cup of coffee has 90 to 150 mg). Table 13.2 lists the chief physical factors to help improve quality of sleep.

RELATIONSHIP OF PHYSICAL ACTIVITY TO SLEEP QUALITY

As indicated in Table 13.2, vigorous exercise should be avoided in the evening, about 4 hours before bed, because this usually increases alertness

TABLE 13.2	Physical Factors for Improving Quality of Sleep
Avoid caffeine 10 h before sleep	
Avoid alcohol and nicotine before sleep	
Avoid heavy meals 1–2 h before sleep	
Avoid exercise 4 h before sleep	
Go to bed and wake up at the same time every day	
Reduce light and noise in the bedroom as much as possible	

in most people. However, regular, vigorous exercise earlier in the day is very helpful in improving quality of sleep. Even moderate aerobic exercise is helpful. For people with insomnia, it is preferable to encourage them to exercise earlier in the day, before dinner, at the latest, to avoid inducing hyperalertness. At least 30 minutes of aerobic exercise—such as walking, bicycling, or jogging—most days of the week, should be the goal. Very slow and gentle exercises to promote muscle relaxation are helpful for most people, after dinner and even immediately before retiring. These might include stretching, yoga (including yoga breathing), or tai chi. A warm bath (not shower) encourages muscle relaxation and may be preferable for people with physical impairments for whom even gentle exercises might be too stimulating immediately before bedtime.

RELATIONSHIP OF DIETARY FACTORS TO SLEEP QUALITY

As indicated in Table 13.2, heavy meals or even a regular meal very close to bedtime may interfere with quality of sleep. Folk wisdom suggests warm milk before bed; since milk is a source of both calcium—which is necessary for muscle relaxation—and tryptophan—which is a precursor to serotonin—there may be some basis for this. Calcium and magnesium deficiencies have been linked to insomnia, so it is important that patients' diets contain the recommended levels of these nutrients. The recommended intake of calcium was increased to 1,000 mg (1,200 mg for women over age 50 and men over age 70 years) in 2010; recommended intake for magnesium is 320 mg daily (see U.S. Department of Agriculture chart at: http://fnic.nal.usda.gov/nal_display/index.php?info_center=4&tax_level=3&tax_subject=256&topic_id=1342&level3_id=5140). Other dietary factors that should be considered as having a negative effect on quality of sleep are skipping meals and/or excessive intake of high-sugar, low-fiber foods. These habits tend to produce imbalances in the blood glucose level and thus act as physiological stressors, triggering the SNS.

COMPLEMENTARY AND ALTERNATIVE MEDICINE APPROACHES TO INSOMNIA

Any complementary therapies that promote muscle relaxation, such as massage therapy, acupuncture, chiropractic and osteopathic manipulation, may be helpful. However, evidence for a direct effect of most Complementary and alternative medicine (CAM) therapies on insomnia is limited at this time.[20,21]

Provider-Based Approaches to Stress Management

Patients with severe psychological stress or those with conditions such as severe hypertension, cardiovascular disease, other serious chronic conditions, and/or depression may need more than self-management techniques to manage stress. Many psychologists specialize in stress management, and can provide much more in-depth supervised training in the self-management approaches described below. Physical approaches to stress management such as yoga and tai chi are often best learned with the assistance of an experienced teacher, especially for patients who have chronic pain, physical disabilities, or who have been sedentary. Clinicians should be sensitive to the patient's possible need for a referral, as appropriate.

Self-Management Approaches

There are a number of evidence-based approaches for self-management of stress. It is best to offer patients several options to increase adherence. All stress management techniques require regular application to be successful; patients must be cautioned that they should not expect immediate results, as they would expect from a medication. Nonpharmaceutical stress management tends to have a gradual but cumulative effect.

The following are effective and popular stress management, or relaxation, techniques that patients can use for self-management:

- Positive self-talk
- Relaxation response (a simple meditation exercise)
- Progressive muscle relaxation
- Autogenic training
- Breathing exercises to balance the autonomic nervous system

CENTRAL CONCEPTS FOR STRESS SELF-MANAGEMENT

To help patients to develop a successful approach to stress management, it is essential to understand several basic issues underlying individuals' response to stress. These are:

1. Control: Feeling out of control of life situations is one of the chief causes of stress. Consequently, successfully managing stress requires that one achieve a sense of control—that is, self-efficacy (see Chapters 2 and 3 for background on this concept). All stress management

techniques involve achieving some type of control—through physical actions, thoughts, and/or breathing rate.

2. Expectations: Almost always, feeling stressed involves negative expectations. Whether these expectations are based on experience, or whether or not they are realistic, is beside the point. Expecting negative consequences and events creates or magnifies the feeling of being stressed. Consequently, stress management techniques involve either establishing neutral expectations, or positive ones. "Learned optimism," a concept associated with Seligman's positive psychology, can contribute to successful stress management by changing the habit of negative expectations.[22]

3. Autonomic nervous system balance: The physiological mechanism that produces the array of symptoms associated with stress is SNS dominance. Thus, decreasing SNS activity is an integral part of stress management. Benson's well-known "relaxation response," in fact, is based on the physiological mechanism for triggering the parasympathetic nervous system (PNS), and counteracting the SNS response.[23,24] It is perhaps indicative of the pervasiveness of stress in modern life that most people have heard of the "fight or flight" response that characterizes activation of the SNS, but few are familiar with the relaxation response, which characterizes activation of the PNS.

We will return to these central issues as we describe how to teach patients to implement several stress management approaches.

POSITIVE SELF-TALK

We all create our world by talking to ourselves as we go about our daily life. Research has found that people who talk to themselves in a positive way—encouraging themselves, approving of themselves, and expecting good things to come their way—have a better quality of life and better overall health.[25]

Positive self-talk (PST) is a type of cognitive behavioral therapy (CBT) in which the individual learns to give himself or herself positive, rather than negative, messages.[26] It is often used with athletes to improve performance, and its basic principles lend themselves to self management.[26] Some concepts from CBT and positive psychology, along with the technique of "positive reframing" discussed in Chapter 3, can promote "learned optimism" in patients, which is very helpful in changing the negative thought processes associated with stress.[22,27]

Cognitive Distortion

The following thought patterns, referred to as cognitive distortions, are characteristic of negative thinking, and if people become aware of them, they can begin to use positive reframing to transform their attitude.[27,28]

- All-or-nothing thinking: Characterized by "always" and "never." "I can never do anything right!" "I always hurt myself when I try to exercise!" One way to correct this is to reframe the thought in the form of a scale: Instead of telling oneself, "That project was a complete disaster!" a person could reframe his or her thoughts by asking, "On a scale of 1 to 10, how successful was my project?" This will move her away from polarized extremes.

- Filtering: Remembering only negative events and filtering out positive ones. A person can correct this by keeping a journal and recording daily events, which will allow him or her to bypass the mental filter that excludes the positive ones.

- Magnification and minimization: Believing that negative events "count" more than positive ones. "I was late to work twice this week so my boss is going to fire me (even though I've never been late before)!" It often helps to ask a trusted friend or relative for a "second opinion" to help gain objectivity in weighing these events.

- "Should" statements: Set rules for your actions and even your emotions: "I shouldn't let things get to me"; "I should always do the right thing." Since "should" always implies judgment, it can be helpful for a patient to list the "should" statement in question, and rephrase it to say what it really means, in specific terms, to him or her—that is, deconstruct it. "I shouldn't let things get to me," might really mean, "I don't know how to deal with multitasking"; or "I'm frustrated because I feel like I have to take care of everyone," or, "Other people will think less of me if I get so emotional." "Should" almost always implies a feeling of inadequacy and a desire to avoid the challenging situation.

Cognitive distortions feed into negative self-talk. Therefore, clinicians can help by using positive reframing while talking with patients. Patients at home, can use this technique on themselves, when they note the occurrence of their habitual negative thought pattern.

Another useful, and perhaps easier, technique is the use of *affirmations*. The patient identifies a focus issue and creates a positive statement "affirming" it. The statement needs to be positive, simple, and stated in the present tense. For example, a patient who is feeling very stressed says, "I just can't take it anymore!" Repeating this message to oneself throughout the day will become a self-fulfilling prophecy. He or she can change this negative self-talk by deciding on an affirmation to replace the negative thought whenever it comes up. It is also important to repeat the affirmation at set times throughout the day, such as upon arising and again before bed. Such an affirmation might be, "I am a strong and resilient woman"; or "I successfully handle whatever comes up."

RELAXATION RESPONSE

Herbert Benson, a Harvard physician, first popularized this term, based on his research in the 1960s to 1980s in eliciting it through biofeedback and Transcendental Meditation.[23,24] It is viewed as the opposite of the SNS response associated with stress, as it triggers the PNS. He developed a

---

The Stress Response

You've probably heard of the "fight or flight" response, which is how your body reacts to stress. Your body reacts to any type of **stress**—physical, mental, or emotional—as if it was an emergency. This causes:
- Blood pressure to increase
- Muscles to tighten
- Breathing to speed up
- Digestion to go slower or even stop
- Mind to get more alert

Your body is not designed to stay on "red alert" all the time! Chronic stress causes health problems.

The Relaxation Response

To get back to being balanced, we need to activate the *opposite* of the stress response: **The relaxation response**. This causes:
- Blood pressure to *decrease*
- Muscles to *relax*
- Breathing to *slow down*
- Digestion to *increase*
- Mind to become *calm*

Research has shown that people can learn to trigger the relaxation response for themselves.

How to Trigger your Relaxation Response

1. Sit in a comfortable position in a quiet place where you won't be disturbed for about 20 min.
2. Close your eyes.
3. Choose a word or phrase that has a strong positive meaning for you. It could be a word from your spiritual tradition, or some other word (e.g., "peace") that is positive and calming. Focusing on this word will replace random thoughts and worries from intruding on your mind.
4. Breathe in slowly and naturally through your nose. Pause a few seconds, then breathe out through your mouth, slowly and without forcing the breath. While you breath out, repeat the focus word silently, in your mind.

Continue for about 10 min; you may want to gradually increase the time to about 20 min.
You may repeat the exercise several times a day, if you wish; at least practice it 3 to 4 times per week.

Figure 13.1. Instructions for the relaxation response. (Data taken from Benson H, Proctor W, *Relaxation Revolution*. New York, NY: Scribner, 2010.)

popular technique to elicit the relaxation response; it is simple, acceptable to a wide range of people, and effective. Figure 13.1 provides instructions to patients for using this technique.

PROGRESSIVE MUSCLE RELAXATION

Progressive muscle relaxation (PMR) is based on the principle that it is very difficult to "try to relax." It therefore focuses on tightening an isolated muscle group, and then letting it go—thus relaxation is automatic rather than a conscious action. One can start at either the head or the feet. Since most people carry a great deal of tension in their upper body, it is often best to start with the head. However, this is an individual choice. Figure 13.2 gives instructions the patient can use to conduct a PMR session. These should be done at least daily. PMR is especially helpful before bed to promote good sleep quality.

AUTOGENIC TRAINING

AT is similar to self-hypnosis. It was developed in the 1930s by Johannes Schultz, a German psychiatrist. He theorized that this method would restore balance to the autonomic nervous system through use of what he termed "formulae."[29] Over the years, AT has been widely used, and a 2008 systematic review demonstrated that it was effective for managing anxiety, which suggests that it would have utility in stress management as well.[30] About 15 minutes per day is recommended, over several months, for an individual to gain competency in AT. Figure 13.3 gives instructions in the basic practice of AT. Additional AT exercises involve calming the heart rate, inducing warmth in the stomach, and coolness in the forehead. Patients should do the heart rate exercise only if the clinician is sure they have no health conditions or do not take any

---

Progressive Muscle Relaxation

We all know how hard it is to "try to relax!" With PMR, you focus instead on *tightening* each muscle— and when you let go, it automatically relaxes. It's called "progressive" because you progress from one group of muscles to another until the whole body becomes relaxed.

Instructions

1. Lie down in a comfortable position on the bed or floor. Be sure the room is quiet and semidark. Be sure your clothing is comfortably loose. Close your eyes.
2. Tighten each area for 5 seconds, and then let it go for a few seconds before you proceed to the next. Experience what it feels like after you let go.
   - Forehead: Pull your eyebrows together, raise them toward the top of your head. Let go.
   - Eyes: Close your eyes tightly, and then open them wide. Let go.
   - Mouth and jaw: Make a snarling face with bared teeth, and then open your mouth as wide as you can. Let go.
   - Hands: Make a fist with both hands at once, and then open your hand, fingers wide apart. Let go.
   - Forearms: Push your hands forward as if pushing against a wall. Let go.
   - Upper arms: Tighten your biceps (upper arms), elbows bent. Let go.
   - Shoulders: Raise your shoulders toward your ears in a shrug. Let go.
   - Back: Arch your lower back. Let go.
   - Abdomen (stomach area): Tighten your lower abdomen, pulling your navel back toward your spine. Let go.
   - Hips: Tighten up your buttock muscles. Let go.
   - Thighs: Push your thighs together. Let go.
   - Feet: Point your toes upward, toward the ceiling, then downward. Let go.
   - Toes: Curl your toes downward, and then spread them apart. Let go.
3. Experience how your body feels now. If any area still feels tense, tighten it and let go again. Repeat as needed.

Figure 13.2. Instructions for progressive muscle relaxation.

Autogenic Training

AT is a self-help technique to help balance your autonomic nervous system. The autonomic nervous system is made up of the SNS and PNS. When you are under stress, your SNS is overactive and produces most of the effects of stress in your body. AT calms your SNS and activates your PNS, which will reduce your stress symptoms.

Lie comfortably with eyes closed on the bed or floor in a semidarkened room. Do each exercise for about a minute, twice a day, for a week before starting the next exercise.

In all the AT exercises, you will be "talking to" your body to train it to relax. You need not talk out loud; repeat the messages silently—you are, after all, talking to yourself! Each exercise uses a different message about an aspect of relaxation.

Exercise 1: Heaviness. Start with your dominant arm (right, if you are right-handed; left, if you are left-handed), then go to the other arm, and then legs.

1) *"My right (left) arm is very heavy."* Repeat 6 times.
2) Follow the heaviness command with, *"I am completely calm."*
3) To return to your normal state, finish session as follows:
   - Make a fist with your hands, then release;
   - Bend and stretch each arm;
   - Take several deep breaths;
   - Open eyes.

Exercise 2: Warmth. First repeat your "heaviness" exercise. Again, start with dominant arm, followed by the other arm and then legs.

1) *My right (left) arm is pleasantly warm.* Repeat 6 times.
2) *"I am completely calm."*
3) To return to your normal state, finish session as follows:
   - Make a fist with your hands, then release;
   - Bend and stretch each arm;
   - Take several deep breaths;
   - Open eyes.

Exercise 3: Calm and Regular Breathing. First briefly repeat your heaviness and warmth exercises.

1) *"My breathing is smooth and quiet."* Repeat 6 times.
2) *"I am completely calm."*
3) To return to your normal state, finish session as follows:
   - Make a fist with your hands, then release;
   - Bend and stretch each arm;
   - Take several deep breaths;
   - Open eyes.

Figure 13.3. Instructions in autogenic training.

medications that might affect the heart. This is the exercise for calming the heart rate:

Exercise: Calm and Regular Heartbeat

Do not do this exercise unless your physician OKs it, if you have or think you may have any heart problems.

4. First repeat your "heaviness" and "warmth" exercises.
5. Give yourself the message *"My heartbeat is calm and regular."* Putting your hand on your chest may help you concentrate. DO NOT try to slow down or speed up your heart rate! Repeat the message six times.
6. Finish with *"I am completely calm."*

Patients should only do the exercise for warming the stomach if the clinician feels it is safe and appropriate. The formula for this exercise is *"Warmth is radiating around my stomach."* The patient should be shown the area on which to focus, since many people have varying concepts of where their stomach is located. Ideally, this exercise triggers the PNS and increases general relaxation.

Finally the "cool forehead" formula is often useful for patients with tension headaches. The formula is, *"My forehead is pleasantly cool."* The patient may wish to imagine a light, cool breeze blowing on the forehead.

BREATHING EXERCISE TO BALANCE THE AUTONOMIC NERVOUS SYSTEM

This technique, based on time-honored yogic breathing practices, is perhaps the simplest and most widely acceptable one for stress management. It requires no belief system and can be done at almost any time and any place. It is based on the simple physiological principle that slow, deep breathing triggers the PNS. Studies have shown that deep, slow breathing slows heart rate and blood pressure, and may also be useful for chronic pain patients.[31–33] The clinician should be sure that the patient has no contraindications to slow breathing, such as severe diabetes, cardiovascular problems, respiratory problems, or hypotension. He or she can be instructed that it is not necessary to attempt to relax or empty the mind; all that is needed is to time one's breathing to 5 to 6 breaths per minute. First be sure the patient uses abdominal breathing. Instructions are provided in Figure 13.4. This exercise is useful for stress in general, but especially for patients with hypertension (if no contraindications are present).

COMMON STRESS-RELATED CONDITIONS: HYPERTENSION AND DEPRESSION

Both hypertension and depression are common conditions and are strongly related to stress, and hence are included in this chapter. However, multiple factors contribute to both hypertension and depression. All the stress management techniques described in this chapter may be helpful for patients with hypertension or depression. However, there are additional important factors to be considered in effectively managing it, and both conditions often require comanagement with several types of providers. The health effects, assessment, and management of these two conditions are described below.

Hypertension
EFFECT OF HYPERTENSION ON HEALTH

It has been estimated that hypertension, defined for adults as systolic blood pressure (SBP) ≥140 mm Hg and diastolic blood pressure ≥90 mm Hg, affects 43 million Americans above age 25 years. Prevalence is higher in African–Americans and in the elderly.[34,35] Hypertension is responsible for 35% of myocardial infarctions and strokes, 49% of episodes of heart failure, and 24% of premature deaths in the United States.[3,35] The risk of stroke, myocardial infarction, heart failure, and peripheral vascular disease is two to four times greater for those with hypertension than those with normal blood pressure.[3,35] End-stage renal disease, retinopathy, and aortic aneurysm are also complications related to hypertension.[3,35]

ASSESSMENT OF HYPERTENSION

Office blood pressure measurement. The standard screening method for hypertension is in-office mercury or aneroid sphygmomanometry using an upper arm cuff. This measure correlates highly with intra-arterial measurement and is also highly predictive of cardiovascular disease risk, when performed correctly.[3,36] However, many errors are possible in routine clinical practice, due to the instrument, the clinician, or the patient.[3,37] To minimize the consequences of such possible errors, hypertension should only be diagnosed after two or more elevated readings at separate visits over a minimum of a 1-week interval.[34]

The Joint National Committee on Prevention, Detection, Evaluation, and Treatment of High Blood Pressure recommends screening intervals

Balance Your Autonomic Nervous System

The autonomic nervous system is made up of the SNS and the PNS. They have opposite functions that balance each other. However, in many people, the SNS is overly active, due to chronic stress. Because functions of the SNS include tensing the muscles, increasing blood pressure, heart rate, and breathing, chronic overactivity of the SNS can result in muscle tension, high blood pressure, and even panic attacks.

This is because the SNS's function is to prepare you to deal with emergencies. Your body perceives stress as a threat and so the SNS is triggered. This is called the *stress response*.

Triggering your PNS produces the opposite: The *relaxation response*.

A simple way to produce the relaxation response is through deep, slow breathing. This automatically triggers the PNS. You don't have to "try to relax," empty your mind of thoughts, or do anything except follow these simple instructions, and your body will simply turn on the PNS:

- Lie down in a comfortable position and loosen your clothing (especially waistband and bra).
- Be sure you have a clock with a second hand at first (later you will not need it once you get accustomed to the breathing rhythm).
- Breathe in through your nose for 5 to 6 s, breathe out through your nose for 5 to 6 s. (This is 5–6 breaths per min, much slower than how you usually breathe). After you have timed yourself a few times, you can dispense with the clock. Some people find counting by saying silently "a thousand and one; a thousand and two . . .") works as accurately as a watch.
- Let your abdomen rise as the breath comes in, but do not raise your shoulders as the breath gets to the top of your lungs. Breathing into the abdomen helps you breathe deeply; raising the shoulders makes you breathe more shallowly.
- Start with 5 min per day; gradually increase to 15 to 20 min per day (5 min at a time, several times a day, will help you stay more relaxed throughout the day).

Figure 13.4. Instructions for how to balance your autonomic nervous system.

of 2 years for people with normal blood pressure (<120/80 mm Hg) and annual screening for those with SBP of 120 to 139 mm Hg or diastolic of 80 to 90 mm Hg.[34]

Home blood pressure monitoring may better assess average blood pressure than does office monitoring, due to the greater number of possible measurements. It is, of course, subject to the same errors in measurement. Definitive evidence is lacking to document its correlation with risks. Therefore, in-office screening remains the standard method to identify hypertension.

EFFECTIVE INTERVENTIONS

Interventions are categorized as pharmacological or nonpharmacological.[3]

Pharmacological Interventions

Medication is effective compared to placebo in reducing cardiovascular events by lowering blood pressure.[34] More than two-thirds of people with hypertension need more than one drug, chosen from different classes, for adequate blood pressure control.[34] Thiazide diuretics are still the more common medication, and have been so since the 1960s. Other classes of drugs are also effective and are currently usually combined with diuretics. These classes are aldosterone receptor blockers (ARBs), angiotensin converting enzyme inhibitors (ACEIs), beta blockers (BBs), and calcium channel blockers (CCBs).[34]

Adverse effects of antihypertensive drugs. "Nonserious" adverse effects are very common in antihypertensive drugs, ranging between 40% and 89% of participants, depending on the study and the particular drug. These include headache, upper respiratory infection, nasopharyngitis, ankle edema, constipation, facial flushing, hyperkalemia, dizziness, and erective dysfunction. Serious adverse effects appear to be less common

(4% to 11% of participants, depending on the study and the drug).[35]

Nonpharmacological Interventions

There is fair to good evidence that specific non-pharmacological treatments reduce cardiovascular events. These interventions are weight reduction in overweight patients, increased physical activity, dietary sodium reduction, potassium supplementation, decreased alcohol intake, and stress management. Reductions in SBP ranged from 3 to 15 mm Hg, varying with the study and type of intervention.[3,34] Table 13.3 summarizes these interventions and their effect on blood pressure. As shown in Table 13.3, stress management is one of the most successful interventions for hypertension. Furthermore, non-pharmacological therapy also appears to be effective for the primary prevention of hypertension.[38]

Depression
EFFECT ON HEALTH

Depression, formally referred to as *major depressive disorder* (MDD), has a lifetime prevalence of 13%.

About 43% of patients in primary care who suffer from MDD report having had suicidal thoughts within the past week.[39] Depression is the number one cause of years of life lived with a disability (YLD). It may increase the risk of physical disability, coronary heart disease, and diabetes mellitus and all-cause mortality. It is a major risk factor for suicide. Depression has significant economic effects, with direct and indirect costs estimated at US $83 billion in 2000.[39]

ASSESSING DEPRESSION STATUS

There is little evidence showing that any one screening tool for depression is better than the others. The U.S. Preventive Services Task Force (USPSTF) recommends these two questions for screening[40]:

"Over the past 2 weeks, have you felt down, depressed, or hopeless?" and

"Over the past 2 weeks, have you felt little interest or pleasure in doing things?"

(A positive answer to either one warrants further assessment.)

TABLE 13.3	Effects of Nonpharmacological Interventions on Systolic Blood Pressure	
Intervention	**Description**	**SBP Reduction (mm Hg)**
Stress management*	Single or multiple component stress management program	9–10
DASH (Dietary Approaches to Stop Hypertension) diet plan	Increase fruits, vegetables, and low-fat dairy products with reduced saturated and total fat	8–14
Weight reduction (overweight/obese)	Maintain BMI 18.5–24.9 kg/m^2	5–20 for 10 kg weight loss
Physical activity	30+ min aerobic exercise, most days of week	4–9
Reduced sodium intake	≤6 g sodium chloride/d	2–8
Alcohol moderation	≤2 drinks per day for men and ≤1 drink per d for women	2–4
Potassium supplementation*	60 meq/d potassium supplementation	3
Tobacco cessation[a]	General	Decreases overall cardiovascular risk

[a]Tobacco cessation decreases overall cardiovascular risk.
BMI, body mass index; SBP, systolic blood pressure.
Source: Unless otherwise specified: From Chobanian AV, Bakris GL, Black HR, et al. Seventh report of the Joint National Committee on Prevention, Detection, Evaluation, and Treatment of High Blood Pressure. Hypertension 2003;42(6):1206–1252, with permission;
* Data taken from Sheridan S, Pignone M, Donahue K. Screening for high blood pressure: a review of the evidence for the U.S. Preventive Services Task Force. *Am J Prev Med.* 2003;25(2):151–158.

Any positive screening test indicates the need for a full diagnostic interview with a trained clinician. Screening alone does not improve the health outcomes for people with depression; it is essential that positive screening be followed up with appropriate case management.[39] Thus, clinicians should have established referral networks for mental health providers and clinics where patients can be referred as needed. Since depression is three to four times more common in people with chronic low back pain than it is in the general population, providers who work with low back pain patients frequently should be especially aware of indications of the presence of depression.[41]

EFFECTIVE INTERVENTIONS

Both psychotherapy and antidepressant medications, alone or in combination, have been shown to be effective in treating depression. The medications considered to be effective are selective serotonin reuptake inhibitors (SSRIs), tricyclic antidepressants (TCAs), and more recently, other non-SSRI "second generation" antidepressants.[39,40]

Adverse effects of antidepressant medications The most important adverse effects noted are (1) increased risk for suicidal behavior (although not actual incidence of suicide) in young adults (ages 18 to 29 years) and (2) increased risk for upper gastrointestinal bleeding in older adults.[39,40]

Physical activity programs involving regular aerobic exercise have also been found to be helpful for managing depression and anxiety.[42,43] Tai chi has also been found to be helpful for depression.[12]

A 2011 meta-analysis found that self-guided treatment for depression, based on Cognitive Behavioral Therapy, had a beneficial effect.[44] However, for patients with clinical depression, it is advisable that providers who work primarily with physical symptoms, especially chronic pain, co-manage the patient with experienced mental health professionals. The stress management techniques described in this chapter may be useful adjuncts for those patients, as well as for patients with mild depression not requiring additional treatment.

Literature Cited

1. American Psychological Association. *Stress in America*. Washington, DC: American Psychological Association; 2007.
2. NIOSH Working Group. *Stress at Work*. Washington, DC: USDHHS; 2011.
3. Sheridan S, Pignone M, Donahue K. Screening for high blood pressure: a review of the evidence for the U.S. Preventive Services Task Force. *Am J Prev Med*. 2003;25(2):151–158.
4. Daubenmier J, Kristeller J, Hecht FM, et al. Mindfulness intervention for stress eating to reduce cortisol and abdominal fat among overweight and obese women: an exploratory randomized controlled study. *J Obes*. 2011;2011:651936.
5. Cohen BE, Panguluri P, Na B, et al. Psychological risk factors and the metabolic syndrome in patients with coronary heart disease: findings from the heart and soul study. *Psychiatry Res*. 2010;175(1–2):133–137.
6. Selye H. *The Stress of Life*. New York, NY: McGraw-Hill; 1956.
7. Anspaugh D, Hamrick, MH, Rosato, FD. *Wellness: Concepts and Applications*. 7th ed. Boston, MA: McGraw-Hill; 2009.
8. Cohen S, Kamarck T, Mermelstein R. A global measure of perceived stress. *J Health Soc Behav*. 1983;24(4):385–396.
9. Holmes TH, Rahe RH. The social readjustment rating scale. *J Psychosom Res*. 1967;11(2):213–218.
10. Kemper K, Bulla S, Krueger D, et al. Nurses' experiences, expectations, and preferences for mind-body practices to reduce stress. *BMC Complement Altern Med*. 2011;11:26.
11. Chiesa A, Serretti A. Mindfulness-based stress reduction for stress management in healthy people: a review and meta-analysis. *J Altern Complement Med*. 2009;15(5):593–600.
12. Wang WC, Zhang AL, Rasmussen B, et al. The effect of Tai Chi on psychosocial well-being: a systematic review of randomized controlled trials. *J Acupunct Meridian Stud*. 2009;2(3):171–181.
13. Wilson SJ, Nutt DJ, Alford C, et al. British Association for Psychopharmacology consensus statement on evidence-based treatment of insomnia, parasomnias and circadian rhythm disorders. *J Psychopharmacol*. 2010;24(11):1577–1601.
14. Roth T. Insomnia: definition, prevalence, etiology, and consequences. *J Clin Sleep Med*. 2007;3(suppl 5):S7–S10.
15. Knutson KL, Van Cauter E, Rathouz PJ, et al. Trends in the prevalence of short sleepers in the USA: 1975–2006. *Sleep*. 2010;33(1):37–45.
16. Luthringer R, Muzet M, Zisapel N, et al. The effect of prolonged-release melatonin on sleep measures and psychomotor performance in elderly patients with insomnia. *Int Clin Psychopharmacol*. 2009;24(5):239–249.

17. Wade AG, Ford I, Crawford G, et al. Nightly treatment of primary insomnia with prolonged release melatonin for 6 months: a randomized placebo controlled trial on age and endogenous melatonin as predictors of efficacy and safety. *BMC Med.* 2010;8:51.

18. Bent S, Padula A, Moore D, et al. Valerian for sleep: a systematic review and meta-analysis. *Am J Med.* 2006;119(12):1005–1012.

19. Garzón C, Guerrero JM, Aramburu O, et al. Effect of melatonin administration on sleep, behavioral disorders and hypnotic drug discontinuation in the elderly: a randomized, double-blind, placebo-controlled study. *Aging Clin Exp Res.* 2009;21(1):38–42.

20. Sarris J, Byrne GJ. A systematic review of insomnia and complementary medicine. *Sleep Med Rev.* 2011;15(2):99–106.

21. Cheuk DK, Yeung WF, Chung KF, et al. Acupuncture for insomnia. *Cochrane Database Syst Rev.* 2007;(3):CD005472.

22. Seligman ME, Csikszentmihalyi M. Positive psychology.An introduction. *Am Psychol.* 2000;55(1):5–14.

23. Hoffman JW, Benson H, Arns PA, et al. Reduced sympathetic nervous system responsivity associated with the relaxation response. *Science.* 1982;215(4529):190–192.

24. Benson H. The relaxation response: history, physiological basis and clinical usefulness. *Acta Med Scand Suppl.* 1982;660:231–237.

25. Sin NL, Lyubomirsky S. Enhancing well-being and alleviating depressive symptoms with positive psychology interventions: a practice-friendly meta-analysis. *J Clin Psychol.* 2009;65(5):467–487.

26. Hamilton R, Miedema B, MacIntyre L, et al. Using a positive self-talk intervention to enhance coping skills in breast cancer survivors: lessons from a community based group delivery model. *Curr Oncol.* 2011;18(2):e46–e53.

27. Burns D. *Feeling Good: The New Mood Therapy.* New York, NY: Avon Books; 1992.

28. Burns DD. *The Feeling Good Handbook: Using the New Mood Therapy in Everyday Life.* New York, NY: William Morrow; 1989.

29. Benson H, Beary JF, Carol MP. The relaxation response. *Psychiatry.* 1974;37(1):37–46.

30. Manzoni GM, Pagnini F, Castelnuovo G, et al. Relaxation training for anxiety: a ten-years systematic review with meta-analysis. *BMC Psychiatry.* 2008;8:41.

31. Zautra AJ, Fasman R, Davis MC, et al. The effects of slow breathing on affective responses to pain stimuli: an experimental study. *Pain.* 2010;149(1):12–18.

32. Pramanik T, Sharma HO, Mishra S, et al. Immediate effect of slow pace bhastrika pranayama on blood pressure and heart rate. *J Altern Complement Med.* 2009;15(3):293–295.

33. Oneda B, Ortega KC, Gusmao JL, et al. Sympathetic nerve activity is decreased during device-guided slow breathing. *Hypertens Res.* 2010;33(7):708–712.

34. Chobanian AV, Bakris GL, Black HR, et al. Seventh report of the Joint National Committee on Prevention, Detection, Evaluation, and Treatment of High Blood Pressure. *Hypertension.* 2003;42(6):1206–1252.

35. Wolff T, Miller T. Evidence for the reaffirmation of the U.S. Preventive Services Task Force recommendation on screening for high blood pressure. *Ann Intern Med.* 2007;147(11):787–791.

36. Reeves RA. The rational clinical examination. Does this patient have hypertension? How to measure blood pressure. *JAMA.* 1995;273(15):1211–1218.

37. McAlister FA, Straus SE. Evidence based treatment of hypertension. Measurement of blood pressure: an evidence based review. *BMJ.* 2001;322(7291):908–911.

38. Whelton PK, He J, Appel LJ, et al. Primary prevention of hypertension: clinical and public health advisory from The National High Blood Pressure Education Program. *JAMA.* 2002;288(15):1882–1888.

39. O'Connor EA, Whitlock EP, Beil TL, et al. Screening for depression in adult patients in primary care settings: a systematic evidence review. *Ann Intern Med.* 2009;151(11):793–803.

40. USPSTF. *Guide to Clinical Preventive Services.* Washington, DC: Agency for Healthcare Research and Quality (AHRQ); 2010.

41. Sullivan MJ, Reesor K, Mikail S, et al. The treatment of depression in chronic low back pain: review and recommendations. *Pain.* 1992;50(1):5–13.

42. Carek PJ, Laibstain SE, Carek SM. Exercise for the treatment of depression and anxiety. *Int J Psychiatry Med.* 2011;41(1):15–28.

43. Lavie CJ, Milani RV, O'Keefe JH, et al. Impact of exercise training on psychological risk factors. *Prog Cardiovasc Dis.* 2011;53(6):464–470.

44. Cuijpers P, Donker T, Johansson R, et al. Self-guided psychological treatment for depressive symptoms: a meta-analysis. *PLoS One.* 2011;6(6):e21274.

CHAPTER 14

Worksite Wellness

Michael Perko

INTRODUCTION

The workplace and the health of the workers are inextricably linked; workplaces should not only protect the safety and well-being of employees but also provide them opportunities for better long-term health and enhanced quality of life. Given that, on an average, Americans working full time spend more than one-third of their day, 5 days per week at the workplace; this is an important setting for health protection, health promotion, and disease prevention programs.

Although employers have a responsibility to provide a safe and hazard-free workplace, they also have abundant opportunities to promote individual health and foster a healthy work environment for more than 139 million workers in the United States.[1] Maintaining a healthier workforce can lower direct costs such as insurance premiums and worker's compensation claims. It will also have a positive impact on many indirect costs such as absenteeism and worker productivity.[2] More importantly, it's the right thing to do.

Helpful definitions of health promotion and wellness are provided in this chapter:

Health Promotion

Health promotion is defined as "any combination of educational and environmental supports for actions and conditions of living conducive to health."[3]

Health promotion is "the process of enabling people to increase control over their health and its determinants, and thereby improve their health."[4]

WORKSITE HEALTH PROMOTION

- "Health is promoted by providing a decent standard of living, good labor conditions, education, physical culture, and means of rest and recreation."[5]
- "The science and art of helping people change their lifestyle to move toward a state of optimal health."[6]

- "An organized program in the worksite that is intended to assist employees and their family members in making voluntary behavior changes that reduce their health risks and enhance their individual productivity and well-being."[7]
- "Worksite health promotion represents a corporate set of strategic and tactical actions that seek to optimize worker health and business performance through the collective efforts of employees, families, employers, communities, and society-at-large."[8]

Wellness

- (The original definition) "An integrated method of functioning, which is oriented toward maximizing the potential of which the individual is capable of functioning within the environment."[9]
- "Wellness is an active process through which people become aware of, and make choices toward, a more successful existence."[10]

WORKSITE WELLNESS

See definitions above for worksite health promotion.

What are Workplace Wellness (WW) programs? WW programs are a coordinated and comprehensive set of strategies, which include programs, policies, benefits, environmental supports, and links to the surrounding community designed to meet the health and safety needs of all employees. They not just a hodgepodge of health activities trying to help employees get healthier; WW is backed by a large scientific evidence base that refers to a coordinated and comprehensive set of tested strategies, which includes programs, policies, benefits, environmental supports, and links to the surrounding community designed to meet the health and safety needs of all employees.

Some examples of WW program components and strategies include:

- Behavior change programs based on evidence-based social science research

- Health education classes
- Incentive programs
- Collaboration with local community partners such as clinicians, to provide value added benefits of employment
- Company policies that promote healthy behaviors such as a tobacco-free setting
- Employee health insurance coverage for appropriate preventive screenings
- A healthy work environment created through actions such as making healthy foods available and accessible through vending machines or cafeterias
- A work environment free of recognized health and safety threats with a means to identify and address new problems as they arise.

SIMPLE BOTTOM LINE

To improve the health of their employees, businesses can (and should) create a wellness culture that is employee-centered, provides supportive environments where safety is ensured and health can emerge, and provides access and opportunities for their employers to engage in various workplace health programs. It's all really about realizing that employees and employers have a symbiotic relationship—the healthiest companies provide access for employees to be at their best. The following sections will provide a short history of worksite health promotion (we will call it worksite wellness here, or WW), the seven benchmarks of America's healthiest companies and finally, provide strategies for clinicians to become part of the WW team in their communities.

HISTORY OF WORKSITE WELLNESS

The concept of employers wanting employees to be healthy is nothing new; one of the first references to employee "exercise" programs was in the 1700s when the following advice was suggested to tailors and cobblers who sat all day, "We shall place among the exercises the movements of the workers and farmers...the strength and good health which peasants enjoy prove to us how much these occupations contribute to life and protect health."[11]

Guldbeck[12] writes that there have been essentially four generations of WW efforts:

1. First generation—any time before the 1950s
2. Second generation—1960s to 1980s
3. Third generation—1990s to present day
4. Fourth generation—still evolving

First-Generation Worksite Wellness

Prior to the 1950s, the scientific literature specifically regarding health and prevention of disease was in its infancy. Therefore, programs in the first generation were not based solely on science but more likely on opportunity and occupational necessity. In the late 1800s, George Pullman, founder of the Pullman Palace Car Company, bought 4,000 acres near Lake Calumet IL, to build the headquarters of his sleeping car company. On this land he built the town of Pullman, adjacent to his factory with its own housing, shopping areas, churches, theaters, parks, hotels, and library for his employees. All Pullman employees lived and worked in Pullman and freely partook in many of the athletic and recreational activities there. According to the Pullman Archive, "Along with being credited with improving the quality of the residents, Pullman was credited with even more miraculous feats, like lowering the death rate." In 1893, Pullman was voted the world's healthiest city.[13] Similarly, in 1894 John Patterson, President of National Cash Register (NCR), took a very measured approach to his employees health. Patterson attributed employees' failure to shabbiness and poor health habits, so NCR provided each shift with clean water for washing, lockers for the employees, and daily coffee. In addition, articles concerning health practices appeared in company publications—these articles instructed employees how to improve their digestion, care for their teeth, and exercise. Other measures included mandatory calisthenics, pre-dawn horseback rides, 10-minute exercise breaks at 10 AM and 3 PM mandated to improve employees' health and efficiency, and in 1902 instituted the Vital Center Physical Culture Course; over 400 men and women employees enrolled in this program.[14] By the turn of the century, as workers left the fields and joined the assembly lines in the era of mass production, first-generation WW programs became much more focused on employee safety, efficiency, and productivity. During the 1930s and 1940s, occupational health and safety programs sought to protect workers from injury, and established guidelines for prevention of on-the-job injuries. One of the first organized WW programs emerged at this time—Texas Instruments formalized an employee recreation and fitness program, and broke ground for an 8-acre fitness facility for employees and their families.[15] Other programs followed, most geared around physical activity and fitness.

Second-Generation Worksite Wellness

From the 1960s to the 1970s, programs in WW began to increase in number and scope, but focused mainly on activities such as walking or tobacco cessation rather than comprehensive programs based on long-term behavior change. The story of Larry Walters can be used here to epitomize WW efforts of the second generation. When Larry Walters was 13 years old, he went to a local Army–Navy surplus store and saw weather balloons hanging from the ceiling. It was then he knew that someday he would be carried aloft by such balloons. This obsession was to be with him for the next 20 years. On July 2, 1982, Larry tied 42 helium-filled balloons to a Sears lawn chair in the backyard of his girlfriend's house in San Pedro, California. With the help of his ground crew, Larry then secured himself into the lawn chair that was anchored to the bumper of a friend's car by two nylon tethers. He took with him many supplies, including a sandwich, some soda pop, and a BB gun to shoot out the balloons when he was ready to descend. His goal was to stay aloft for a few hours with a great view. But things didn't quite work out for Larry. After his crew cut the first tether, the second one suddenly snapped, which shot Larry into the LA sky at over 1,000 feet per minute. So fast was his ascent that he lost his glasses. He then climbed to over 16,000 feet. For several hours, he drifted in the cold air near the LA and Long Beach airports. A commercial airline pilot first spotted Larry and radioed the tower that he was passing a guy in a lawn chair at 16,000 feet! Larry started shooting out a few balloons to start his descent but had accidentally dropped the BB gun. He eventually landed in a Long Beach neighborhood. Although he was entangled in some power lines, he was uninjured. The story of Larry Walter captures WW programs in the second generation—they seemed like a good idea at the time and everyone was behind them; once they got going, however, no one knew where they were going or where they would end.

The early second-generation WW programs were characterized by a narrow focus on one method of delivery such as only in a fitness center, a single illness or risk factor, for example heart disease, or programs offered to only one population like CEO's. Emerging data at this time coming from the Framingham Study,[16] the Surgeon General's Report on Smoking and Health,[17] and the growing field of exercise science began to show that changes in behavior could reduce risk for both acute and chronic illness. The first systematic effort at risk reduction rather than simple recreation was attempted during the second generation; however, many of these efforts focused on keeping senior management healthy; oftentimes the general employee population did not have access to the company facilities. Various psychosocial theories began to be applied to WW programs and a body of scientific evidence to support much more comprehensive WW programs began in earnest. In 1977 the National Wellness Institute (NWI) in Stevens Point, Wisconsin held its first conference to bring together WW directors and practitioners to discuss the "state of the art" in WW. Universities began to offer coursework and degrees in worksite health promotion, and textbooks exploring all aspects of WW were available. Since the 1980s, four national surveys of WW programs have been conducted; results show with each survey that more and more companies are offering WW programs for their employees. The first national survey of worksite health promotion activities in the United States was conducted in 1985 (with follow-up surveys conducted in 1992, 1999, and 2004); results showed that of 1,358 American companies, 65% were offering at least one WW program or activity.[18] Program activities included smoking cessation, fitness, weight management, back problem prevention and care, and stress management. Participation typically was the metric most cited as having successful programs; programs that utilized evaluation data based on more complex metric measures such as absenteeism and productivity were rare.

Third-Generation Worksite Wellness

Worksite wellness programs in the third generation have grown in sophistication with a greater emphasis on policy changes to support healthful environments, program evaluation, and return on investment (ROI). The singular focus on program activities of the second generation have given way to more broad, comprehensive, and outcomes-based programs. Accordingly, the 2010 Healthy People Report[19] included the five objectives needed in WW for a program to be considered comprehensive:

- Health Education programs,
- Supportive social and physical environments,
- Integration of the program into the organizational structure,
- Linkages to related programs such as Health and Safety and Employee Assistance Programs (EAP), and
- Worksite Screenings

National surveys continue to show great interest in WW by companies and that trend should continue as a strategic initiative to contain future healthcare costs. Clear evidence shows that WW can save money by delaying or reducing risk among an employee population. A 1998 review of early WHP studies, mostly conducted in the 1980s and early 1990s,[20] estimated ROI savings ranging from US $1.40 to US $3.14 per dollar spent, with a median ROI of ~ US $3.00 saved per dollar spent on the program. In 2001, Aldana[21] performed a comprehensive literature review of the financial impact of health promotion programming on health care costs in which he rated the rigor of the evaluations. Only 4 of 32 studies reviewed reported no effects of health promotion on health care costs. However, these four studies did not employ a randomized design, whereas several of the other studies that reported positive results applied experimental or rigorous quasi-experimental methods. The average ROI for seven studies reporting costs and benefits was US $3.48 for every dollar expended. In 2005, Chapman summarized results from 56 qualifying financial impact studies conducted over the previous two decades and concluded that participants in worksite programs have 25% to 30% lower medical and absenteeism costs compared with nonparticipants, over an average study period of 3.6 years.[22] Some might argue that rising health care costs have caused organizations to see employees only as "future costs" and the singular focus on ROI model has left out the very complex nature of behavior and behavior change. In fact, as we will see in the proposed fourth generation of WW, a refocus on employee's needs, interests, and wants that allow them to achieve personal wellness goals will better serve the organization and still achieve the valued ROI.

Fourth-Generation Worksite Wellness

Chapman[7] proposed what could be described as a prototypical fourth-generation WW model by incorporating both organizational, health, and productivity management that includes the following components integrated together:

- Population Management Focused
- Culture/Climate-based
- Stakeholder Owned/Driven
- Integrated Program Mix
- Multidisciplinary Team
- Align with Benefits Plan
- Intervention Focus
- Coach/Counsel Model

- Motivational Interviewing
- Individual/Group Tailoring
- High Technology Tools
- Health Cost Management/Productivity Metrics

The mind set of fourth-generation WW is that employee health cannot be separated from the strategic mission and purpose of the organization. With fourth definition WW in mind, this is a good place to introduce another definition, this one provided by Michael O'Donnell, editor-in-chief of the American Journal of Health Promotion. "Health Promotion is the art and science of helping people discover the synergies between their core passions and optimal health, enhancing their motivation to strive for optimal health, and supporting them in changing their lifestyle to move toward a state of optimal health.[23]

As the field moves toward fourth-generation WW, what we know for sure is that:

1. Worksite wellness programs can lead to positive changes at both the individual (i.e., employee) and the organization levels.
2. For individuals, worksite wellness programs have the potential to impact an employee's health, such as their health behaviors; health risks for disease; and current health status.
3. For organizations, worksite wellness programs have the potential to impact areas such as health care costs, absenteeism, productivity, recruitment/retention, culture, and employee morale.
4. Employers, workers, their families, and communities all benefit from the prevention of disease and injury and from sustained health.
5. Current and future legislative actions including health reform stress prevention at all levels—this will induce more companies to explore WW as a health strategy.

SEVEN KEY BENCHMARKS OF SUCCESSFUL PROGRAMS

There is no doubt that WW is seen as a strong strategic business investment that can save lives and money; in fact, over 90% of companies in America offer at least one WW activity.[31] The specter of Larry Walters however hangs over many of these programs. Without thoughtful planning, appropriate resources, support at all organizational levels, and documentation of outcomes, WW can be seen as just a line item, so if and when times get tough, program resources are cut. How do the best programs survive, year after year? The Wellness Council of America (WECOA), a national leader in WW program support, has identified seven key benchmarks[25] which, when present, help programs succeed over potential challenges. The following section will provide a synopsis of these benchmarks.

Benchmark 1—Capturing CEO Support

Multiple best practices point to CEO support being the most essential benchmark in the process of developing and maintaining long-term result-based wellness programs. Strong evidence suggests that programs that have contained costs and improved employee health have strong senior-level support.

Benchmark 2—Creating a Cohesive Wellness Team

Once CEO support has been secured, creating a cohesive wellness team helps to distribute the responsibility for wellness through multiple organizational levels. It also allows for continuity when wellness team members, including directors, leave, retire, or get reassigned. The best companies do not rely on just one "wellness person" to run the show—if he or she were to leave the company or retire, the WW program could disband.

Benchmark 3—Collecting Data to Drive Health Efforts

Evidence-based wellness programming dictates that the first primary step in program development is not to start offering programs, but rather to step back and gather data from multiple sources internal to the organization. Data collected using corporate culture audits, health risk appraisals, and knowledge and interest surveys will allow for strategic planning in both organizational business needs and employee interests.

Benchmark 4—Carefully Crafting an Operating Plan

After data is collected, the task is now to develop an operating plan for health and wellness within the organization. This operating plan serves as the roadmap and will guide the company's efforts and investments in WW.

Benchmark 5—Choosing Appropriate Interventions

With the first four benchmarks completed, it is now appropriate to begin choosing and implementing the appropriate health and productivity interventions. These interventions will most likely include tobacco cessation, physical activity, weight management, self-care, and stress management. But, they also may include things like fatigue management, ergonomics, and so on, depending on what the company's data reveals.

Benchmark 6—Creating a Supportive Environment

To coincide with appropriate health promoting interventions, creation of supportive environments will ensure increased participation and compliance. Evidence shows that by having a supportive environment, organizations can be confident that employees will be supported in their efforts to lead healthier lives. Environmental interventions may take the form of policies, physical modifications, and rewards and incentives.

Benchmark 7—Carefully Evaluating Outcomes

The seventh and final benchmark in the WW model is carefully evaluating outcomes. The best companies document outcomes and establish procedures to improve all aspects of the wellness program. Evaluation targets include participation, participant satisfaction, biometric changes, behavior modification, cost containment, and ROI.

ENTRY POINTS FOR CLINICIANS TO BECOME ENGAGED IN WORKSITE PROGRAMS

Although many companies use in-house employees to administer WW programs, there are multiple integration points for partnering with community resources including health professionals that can help take WW programs to world class levels. The following will highlight some of the entry points that should be explored.

Team Member

Health professionals from the local community bring expertise to the table when included as part of a company's WW team. Often WW teams rely on in-house resources to serve employees—the best teams seek out local resources and partner with college and university faculty and students, cooperative extension program staff, and the medical community such as nurses, clinicians, hospital staff, and so on. A key strategy to engage local companies is to participate in yearly health screenings and provide services in kind as a local community member.

Health and Safety Expertise

Injury prevention and safety are two leading areas where clinicians can positively engage local WW programs. Many companies' cultures embrace safety as a core value; providing expertise as a seminar speaker, demonstrations of injury preventions techniques, and ergonomic evaluation are all highly valued contributions to WW programming.

Health Content Expert

Giving accurate health information via talks or seminars is a fundamental component of WW programs. The training and experience of the clinicians makes them valuable allies to companies who want to give accurate and appropriate information to employees.

Health Biometric Screening Vendor

Health screenings are annual events that draw large numbers of employees. Providing appropriate clinical services to employees can help build long-term relationships with companies.

Nutrition and Fitness Consultation

With 8 of the 10 leading causes of death caused by preventable behaviors, providing consultation in areas such as nutrition, weight control, and fitness can provide employees with the required expert services and allow clinicians to become valuable members of a company's goal for healthier employees (and healthier communities).

Wellness Consultant/Contractor

Innovations in WW delivery, emerging research, and strategic planning can task even the best directors of these programs. Many WW program directors do not manage these programs full time so look for outside consultants to provide expertise and direction. Consultants can be hired on an ad hoc basis charging by the hour for their services, or can contract out several hours per week in a long-term arrangement. Working with multiple companies can provide extra visibility to help lead these programs in addition to increased revenue.

SUMMARY

History was made when in March 2010, when Congress passed the health care bill and the President signed into law the Affordable Care Act.

The Affordable Care Act included the creation of a Prevention Fund, established to provide communities around the country with more than US $16 billion over the next 10 years to invest in effective, proven prevention efforts; including worksite wellness. With this comes a paradigm shift in the way Americans, and American businesses, approach health care. As a result, the WW trend will continue as a strong business strategy in which companies reinvest in their employees' health.

Literature Cited

1. U.S. Bureau of Labor Statistics. http://www.bls.gov/ces/cesprog.htm#Data_Available. Accessed March 14, 2012.
2. Naydeck BL, Pearson JA, Ozminkowski RJ, et al. The impact of the highmark employee wellness programs on 4-year healthcare costs. *J Occup Environ Med.* 2008;50(2):146–156.
3. Green LW, Kreuter MW. *Health promotion planning: an educational and ecological approach,* 3rd ed. Mountain View, CA: Mayfield; 1999:27.
4. World Health Organization. The Bangkok Charter for Health Promotion in a Globalized World (11 August 2005). 6th Global Conference on Health Promotion. 2005. http://www.who.int/healthpromotion/conferences/6gchp/bangkok_charter/en/index.html. Accessed May 30, 2011.
5. Sigerist HE. *The University at The Crossroads: Addresses & Essays.* New York, NY: Henry Schuman; 1946:127.
6. O'Donnell MP. Definition of health promotion. *Am J Health Promot.* 1986;1(1):4–5.
7. Chapman LS. *Planning Wellness.* Seattle, WA: Chapman Institute: 2007:213.
8. The International Association for Worksite Health Promotion. Atlanta announcement on *Worksite Health Promotion,* March 26, 2009. http://www.acsm-iawhp.org/files/Atlanta-Announcement.pdf. Accessed June 16, 2011.
9. Dunn H. High-level wellness for man and society. *Am J Public Health Nations Health.* 1959; 49(6):786–792. http://www.ncbi.nlm.nih.gov/pmc/articles/PMC1372807/. Accessed June 16, 2011.
10. National Wellness Institute. Defining wellness. http://www.nationalwellness.org/index.php?id_tier=2&id_c=26. Accessed June 24, 2011.
11. Shephard RJ. A short history of occupational fitness and health promotion. *Prev Med.* 1991;20(3):436–445.
12. Goldbeck WB, Foreword. In: O'Donnell MP, Ainsworth TH, eds. *Health Promotion*

in the Workplace. John Wiley & Sons, Inc. 1984:v–viii.

13. Pullman Archives. http://www.pullmanil.org/links.htm. Accessed May 26, 2011.

14. Schleppi JR. "It Pays": John H. Patterson and industrial recreation at the National Cash Register Company. *J Sport Hist*. 1979;6(3):20–28

15. Chenoweth DH. *Worksite Health Promotion*, 2nd ed. Champaign, IL: Human Kinetics; 2007.

16. Dawber TR, Moore FE, Mann GV. Coronary heart disease in the Framingham study. *Am J Public Health Nations Health*. 1957;47(4 Pt 2):4–24.

17. The Reports of the Surgeon General. The 1964 Report on Smoking and Health. http://profiles.nlm.nih.gov/NN/Views/Exhibit/narrative/smoking.html. Accessed June 21, 2011.

18. Fielding JE, Piserchia PV. Frequency of worksite health promotion activities. *Am J Public Health*. 1989;79(1):16–20.

19. U.S. Department of Health and Human Services. *Healthy People 2010: With Understanding and Improving Health and Objectives for Improving Health*. 2nd ed. Washington, DC; 2000.

20. Chapman LS. Meta-evaluation of worksite health promotion economic return studies: 2005 update. *Am J Health Promot*. 2005;19(6):1–11.

21. Aldana SG. Financial impact of health promotion programs: a comprehensive review of the literature. *Am J Health Promot*. 2001;15(5):296–320.

22. Goetzel RZ, Juday TR, Ozminkowski RJ. *What's the ROI? A Systematic Review of Return-On-Investment (ROI) Studies of Corporate Health And Productivity Management Initiatives*. AWHP's Worksite Health; 1999: 6:12–21.

23. O'Donnell, MP. Definition of health promotion 2.0: embracing passion, enhancing motivation, recognizing dynamic balance, and creating opportunities. *Am J Health Promot.*, 2009;24(1):iv.

24. Linnan L, Bowling M, Childress J, et al. Results of the 2004 National Worksite Health Promotion Survey. *Am J Public Health*. 2008;98(8):1503–1509.

25. The Wellness Council of America (WELCOA). Activity-Centered Vs. Results-Oriented worksite wellness programs. 2009. http://www.welcoa.org/wellworkplace/index.php?category=2. Accessed June 12, 2011.

CHAPTER 15

Retooling Your Office for Health Promotion and Wellness

Marion W. Evans Jr.

Today it is common to see the words "wellness clinic" or "wellness" used as part of the title on a clinic sign. This can be seen on all sorts of medical and health care offices and in some cases, nonmedical businesses such as health food stores or spa. To most consumers, wellness is probably associated with health care in some capacity. However, what happens if your clinic or center name has "wellness" in it but you don't really have an office plan conducive to delivery of the services the name implies? Although this book is meant to serve as a guide to services you might include in a wellness- or prevention-oriented practice, each practitioner will have to determine which services are feasible in his or her own office. Some services can be provided in the office and some services, such as health screenings, may have to be referred to another provider. It is a good idea to think about what you can and want to offer in your office. Once you are done with that your office materials should reflect what you offer or accent those services. Your goal should be to implement a system to detect modifiable risk factors in patients through lifestyle or behavior change and to prevent disease from occurring prematurely, wherever this is possible.

Signage that indicates the availability of wellness services in the clinic must be supported by what patients experience once they walk through the doors. For example, if yours is truly a wellness clinic, each new patient is likely to be screened for risk factors for premature onset of disease. Your intake paperwork, history, review of systems forms, and diagnostic procedures must include the necessary items to complete a true assessment of the patient's current health status.

PATIENT INTAKE PAPERWORK

Intake paperwork includes the information the patient provides you when he or she first arrives as a new patient or as a reactivated patient. This form can serve as a forum to ask questions related to risk. For instance, do you have check boxes that appear beside the term "smoker" and "nonsmoker"? If so, a wellness practice would also want to include at that level of intake the terms, "former smoker," "other tobacco use," "how many years," and "how many packs per day." It may also be appropriate to have the category of, "former smoker" because some will identify themselves as former smokers rather than nonsmokers. The category for nonsmoker may be most appropriately labeled "never smoked." This reduces the chance of a former smoker who has successfully stopped smoking to self-categorize as a nonsmoker. There is a difference in the health risks of former smokers as compared to those who have never smoked, as tobacco use of any kind has some degree of associated risk. Not all of these health risks subside if the patient quits smoking, so this variability in current status is important to note.

Intake forms should ask about other possible lifestyle related risks as well. The forms can include questions about how many servings of fruits and vegetables are consumed by the patients each day, how many minutes do they exercise each week, or even how they perceive their current stress levels. This author had a section once that asked:

- Are you interested in pain relief only today?
- Are you interested in pain relief and preventing your problem from reoccurring?
- Or are you interested in pain relief, prevention of reoccurrence, and improving your overall personal health?

Most patients chose the third option but many chose pain relief only. It helps to know your patient's current state of readiness for change. This may change with time but early on, you can benefit from knowing their frame of mind; but you have to ask.

Patient History

In the history section of your patient evaluation, it is critical to know the family history, as many will have a history that predisposes them to early on-set of disease. Cardiovascular disease (CVD) is an example. Although the patients can change their lifestyle and perhaps reduce this risk, the fact that an immediate family member had or has CVD increases the risk of them developing it. Although it may seem obvious to suggest that the history include family medical history, the author has seen offices where it was not included.

In the current medical history of the patient, it is not only a good idea to inquire about medications being taken, but to ask about all pills, supplements, vitamins, and herbs. There are two important reasons for this: (1) Some do not consider a pill they take every day (such as a diuretic) to be a medicine. It's just a pill they have taken every day for years! (2) Today it is common for people to self-medicate with herbs or vitamins and minerals, and this can tip you off diagnostically to a potential health ailment they may have that could respond to lifestyle changes. In some cases, it may make you aware of a condition they have not reported to a health care provider at all. In addition, some of these "natural" substances also have side effects or interactions that you may want to know about such as limiting platelet aggregation in the case of garlic or fish oils. Sometimes assessment of health status can include actions taken by patients that they think are helpful but which really put them at greater risk.

In the current medical history section it is important to dig a little regarding health problems the patients may have experienced. Are any of these problems amenable to increased physical activity, dietary change, or other lifestyle changes? This is where the wellness evaluation starts. It is important to ascertain whether there is a health issue that is keeping them from being physically active or if they are having issues maintaining a healthy diet. In this new paradigm, we are not only interested in what is symptomatic but what can be done through behavior change to reduce the risks a patient has or how we can return them to activity, a healthier diet, or safer lifestyle. You will probably start asking more questions.

With any early assessment of a patient related to possible preventive efforts, some will not be ready to make a lifestyle change. A patient who has high cholesterol may prefer to take a pill and not increase physical activity or change his or her diet. But that doesn't mean you should not assess their desire to make positive lifestyle changes. It is likely that no other clinician has ever advised them to make a change in their routine and the pill is the only thing prescribed.

Within your section on history it is very important today to assess surgical history. Although this may not seem relevant to wellness and health promotion, or to behavior change, present day's bariatric procedures can assist a patient in reducing the risk of morbid obesity. Some may have had this surgery performed and it should be a part of the new wellness history as rapid changes in weight can be seen with these procedures. You will want to do everything possible to help patients stay the course, even if surgery has been helpful initially. Lifestyle changes are a lifelong process.

A complete history also includes alcohol use, sexual history, and history of infections. Alcohol screenings can be as simple as asking how many times in the previous year have they consumed over five drinks in one sitting.[1] Infectious disease history is also important as in the case of methicillin-resistant *Staphylococcus aureus* (MRSA), a risk factor includes previous history of MRSA.[2] And this bug seems to be showing up everywhere; including private clinical offices.[3–4]

It is important to remember to ask age-appropriate questions in the history. You probably don't need to ask a 9-year-old about their alcohol history in most cases; however, there could be exceptions. Think about the risks most likely for a specific age group and ask questions that are likely to identify them in your patient based on their age. One should not rule out risks simply based on age, but you should at least formulate an idea of what is most likely based on this demographic variable. If your nurse or staff handles intake paperwork, be sure to have them flag a patient's chart when there are modifiable risk factors that should be addressed. This can be done with a post-it note, a highlighter, or even a colored tape tab available at most office supply stores. Some training of staff may be required to have them move toward a preventive mindset in the office. Start with having them assist you and flag behavioral risk factors.

Review of Systems

The review of systems is often taken for granted. In this situation you will go over each organ or bodily system and see if the patients have a history of current and/or past issues with their health in any of these areas. You should be thinking about how many past or current health conditions could be improved with lifestyle modification. Are there any that need screenings performed or updated? If so, make a note to mention this in your report of findings to the patient. The United States Preventive Services Task Force (USPSTF) has a document listing all recommended screenings and can be a valuable reference.[5]

In the case of a review of systems, if you have a smoker, for example, who states he has some health issues possibly related to tobacco use, it is appropriate to ask him if he has ever made a quit attempt. You may wish to "advise" the patient on cessation later but it is pertinent to know if he has a successful history of cessation. Many smokers have quit in the past but for whatever reason, have started to smoke again. The same can be said for weight loss. However, most of your findings from the history and review of systems can wait until you have examined the patient and are going to report your findings related to what you can do for their condition or improvement of their health.

PATIENT EXAMINATION

Every provider has a routine they perform with patients. Your staff or nurse may take vital signs or perhaps, you don't take them. If your intent is to provide wellness and health promotion in your practice, let's agree that vital signs will be taken on every new patient and every reactivation. If you have patients with a history of hypertension that you see periodically, please take their blood pressure every time they come in. You never know when it may be elevated unless you check it. And it only takes a couple of minutes! Make sure your examination covers everything you can possibly cover that may detect a preventable disease or may detect the need to intervene in a health situation to reduce a threat or harm. You may wish to incorporate a health risk appraisal instrument. Health risk appraisals (HRAs) are common in prevention environments. They can be a part of your routine evaluation. The SF-36 is a series of questions that can score a patient's overall health status.[6] There are also several good HRAs available online. You could have your patient visit a Website while in your office or even outside of your office visit and complete an HRA. He or she could then generate a printout, since many online programs will allow this, and bring it in on his or her next visit for your review. These will typically identify most modifiable risk factors and some that are not modifiable, such as genetic history. However, those that can be addressed should be identified. Table 15.1 lists some sources of online HRAs that you may find of value for your patient.

HRAs should help you assign risks based on age, gender, and other behavioral characteristics. For example, in a younger patient, failure to wear seat belt, speeding when driving, and other increased risk of unintentional injury may be paramount when you see the results of their HRA, whereas in older patients it will be risks for chronic disease. Some younger patients will also have these risks based on tobacco use or family history but it is important to note the risks will break down along demographic lines and this includes age.

Report of Findings

Once you have reviewed intake paperwork, history, review of systems, and examined your patients, they are ready to hear your report of findings (ROF). The ROF is where you must tell them the good, the bad, and the ugly. Hopefully, this also includes the modifiable. We have discussed types of communication skills you need to employ earlier in the text. You will use your authority as a clinician to tell them what they need to do, both with respect to treatment and to lifestyle, to restore their health or treat their condition. Remember, you can state, "As your doctor

TABLE 15.1 Health Risk Appraisal Instruments	
University of Wisconsin–Stevens Point Lifescan	http://wellness.uwsp.edu/other/lifescan
HealthStatus.com	http://www.healthstatus.com
Mayo Clinic	http://www.mayoclinichealthsolutions.com/products/Health-Assessment.cfm
Real Age	http://www.realage.com
American Heart Association–Heart Attack Risk Calculator	https://www.heart.org/gglRisk/locale/en_US/index.html?gtype=health
National Heart Lung and Blood Institute (NHLBI)	http://www.nhlbi.nih.gov/health/public/heart/obesity/lose_wt/risk.htm

or provider . . . it is important to your health that you make change X . . ." or, to adhere to a treatment regimen. However, you should mention the things they may have to address in their lifestyle to get better. If appropriate, let them know you do not expect them to do this right now but perhaps when they are out of pain or no longer sick. But if it is something they should start today, tell them to start today. For example, many painful conditions are not exacerbated by exercise, as long as it is not strenuous or contraindicated by the health history. If they need to start walking every day, it's OK to tell them to start today.

Assisting in initiating any new behavior change process is encouragement, information, and a direct plan of attack. You can call it a lifestyle prescription if you want. Gain-frame the message by telling them what positives will the new change bring about, rather than the negatives such as, you will be sore tomorrow or you will die prematurely if you don't do this. Gain-framing, as explained in Chapter 4, states the benefits of the new behavior rather than the dangers of the old.

RESOURCES

It is important to have resources available if you expect a patient to commit and become successful at behavior changes. This is particularly so if you do not directly provide the instruction or enhancement of skills in your office, which is often the case. Who is your smoking cessation person? Do you have a Lung Association program or a hospital nearby that has a good program? Larger cities will have lists of all of the programs that can be found on a Google search of smoking cessation programs. The goal here is that the patient needs to leave with the information in hand on his or her first visit (or on the day you advise the behavior change), along with directions on how to get started. Do you have a preferred fitness person, gym, dietician, yoga instructor, massage therapist, and psychologist? If so, you may want to have their business card on hand. Feel free to make a referral call or have your front desk person do this for them before they leave your office. This may be the extra touch that will motivate the patient to attempt a behavior change. After all, many patients have never had their health care provider initiate a preventive action, so this may seem novel to them. Take advantage and strike while the iron is hot.

Do you have good, stage-based brochures on tobacco cessation, diet, and needed physical activity? These brochures are often freely available at places like the Centers for Disease Control and Prevention (CDC), the American Public Health Association (APHA), and National Cancer Institute (NCI). Many are available for download, and you can print one out and hand it to your patient. What about DVDs or books to lend? If this is something you want to do, build that library and develop a system to track what you lend out or you may never see it again. Many medical journals or even Medscape and related sites have flyers on various positive health behaviors that are open copyright, so that you can copy them and give them to patients. Having a file cabinet dedicated to materials you want to use to promote positive behavior change is a good idea, and you can keep several of your favorite topics copied and stored in the file cabinet for easy distribution. You can also create your own self-help topics and make forms on your PC or MAC that tell your patients step-by-step what they can do to make a positive change. For example, you might have a sheet on, *"Three Things You Can Do Today to Feel Better Sooner?"* or something similar to provide to each new patient. You can decide the three things based on the type of practice you have. And it gives a personal touch to include your office name and logo and provide a refrigerator magnet. Plus, their friends will see it too! Focusing on the 10 Leading Health Indicators may be a helpful place to start. Table 15.2 lists these from the *Healthy People* Website.

Posters in your treatment room that promote healthy diet, tobacco cessation, physical activity, and wearing seatbelts can be a nice addition to art work and medical charts. While patients are

TABLE 15.2	Ten Leading Health Indicators

Physical activity
Overweight and obesity
Tobacco use
Substance abuse
Responsible sexual behavior
Mental health
Injury and violence
Environmental quality
Immunization
Access to health care

Source: From http://www.healthypeople.gov/2010/LHI/ (This site is an archived site as the new HP 2020 site is active. However, the leading health indicators from HP 2010 in many cases are areas that clinicians can focus on in practice), with permission.

waiting, why not have an informational poster on what tobacco cessation will do or how to get more physical activity? These can be found free of charge from various sources or purchased for a modest price. Frame them with some inexpensive frames if you prefer.

Toolkit

In addition to HRAs, you can find computerized body mass index (BMI) calculators and other instruments online. The CDC has an easy to use BMI calculator available at: http://www.cdc.gov/healthyweight/assessing/bmi/adult_bmi/english_bmi_calculator/bmi_calculator.html. This calculator is for adults because BMI for children uses a formula based on height and weight and their percentile for age. You can find one for children on the CDC site as well. While Table 10.1 contains information on adult BMI, Table 15.3 provides the different BMI categories for children based on percentiles for age/weight. If you treat children, be sure to differentiate them from the adult scale and use the children's method of calculating. For example, an adult is considered overweight with a BMI of 30 or higher, while a male child of 10 years would be considered overweight with a BMI of 21 based on child BMI methodology.[7]

Your tool kit can include anything to help patients make behavioral changes. Forms such as the behavior change contract can be copied in advance. You may want to use a prescription pad to prescribe a lifestyle change or have copies of handouts in racks near the front office that can be picked up for free. It is also a good idea to have free literature in your treatment rooms so a person can take a few when

no one is looking. Why not? This is the goal, right?

Tools can be people, other health care professionals, and instruments you may use to measure body fat percentage such as bio-impedance, calipers, spirometers, blood pressure cuffs in each room, visual analog scales from 0 to 10 related to how ready they are to make a change, and even a room where they can watch a short DVD on how to get motivated. It's really up to you.

HEALTH BEHAVIORAL CONTRACTS

Some clinicians like to use health behavioral contracts. This is a simple document that spells out what you expect the patient to do on the basis of an agreed upon plan established collaboratively between the two of you. Remember, this is a partnership and people resist what they do not help plan. Once you agree on, for example, three things the patient will work on between now and the next visit, list them and get both the doctor and patient to sign the document. Place a copy in the patient file and send one home with a refrigerator magnet so he can display it at home. It could be as simple as agreeing that the patient will walk for 15 minutes, 4 days a week over the next week and that he or she will receive a call from the office to check up on his or her progress on Wednesday afternoon. The copy then gets signed by both and the date is entered on it. The form can have your clinic name and logo, a space for listing the targeted behavior, and the follow-up date as well.

CHARTING BEHAVIOR CHANGE

Although it goes without saying that you must chart anything you suggest in the office, we will say it here for emphasis. Chart what you tell your patient as you would any other recommendation or treatment procedure. This is a part of your care and you must document it. If you have a behavior change contract, place a copy in the file. If you plan to follow-up next visit, make a note in the chart that says, "Ask Mrs. Smith about her walking plan." Highlight it, add a post-it note or whatever other method you prefer that will remind you to ask. Even put a note by the patient's name in the appointment book. The idea is not to let the next visit go by without asking about progress. The last thing you want to do here is recommend a change and not follow-up the next time you see the patient. Have a plan for follow-up. This is critical.

TABLE 15.3	Body Mass Index and Percentiles in Children
Category[a]	**Percentile Range (BMI for Age/Weight)**
Underweight	<5th
Healthy weight	5th to <85th
Overweight	85th to <95th
Obese	≥95th

BMI, Body Mass Index
[a]Body fat composition changes over the child's formative years, so BMI is based on percentiles rather than firm categorization.
Source: From http://www.cdc.gov/healthyweight/assessing/bmi/childrens_bmi/about_childrens_bmi.html, with permission.

THE WELLNESS OFFICE VIBE

How does your office look and feel? Does it only have sports and women's magazines in the reception area? How about a copy of *Prevention* or *Men's Health*? Your literature or lack thereof related to health and wellness makes a statement about your wellness philosophy. You and your staff should perform a walk-through and see if what you currently do reflects a wellness and prevention practice or simply symptomatic care. Do you have living plants or plastic? Is there a spring water cooler in your hallway or do you have patients rely on the cola machine next door? Each of these makes a statement about you and what your office believes about health. If staff are allowed to eat their Big Mac and fries at the front desk while patients are checking in, this might send a mixed signal to the patient you are about to ask to exercise more and reduce fried foods.

Some clinicians are beginning to offer natural supplements in their practices. Although we make no judgment either way on whether you should or should not do this, we caution health care providers about the use of products that make unsubstantiated claims, are unregistered products, or rely on multilevel type of marketing plans that may be unethical in a clinical setting. If you routinely recommend vitamin D for instance, it would seem reasonable to have it available in your office or recommend a local health food store or drug store who stocks a particular reputable brand. However, unproven, gimmicky products should be avoided and discouraged. Patient-centered wellness care is about what is in the best interest of the patient. Concerning nutritional supplements, if you want to check a brand you wish to recommend or, a product your patient is taking, go to www.consumerlab.com and you will be able to find reputable brands along with the not-so-reputable. While you have to subscribe to have full access, the cost is affordable. You may also want to recommend this site to patients as you can become a member of the site and have 24/7 access to check brands and products for ingredients and safety. The site reviews hundreds of products and brands on a regular basis and informs users of deficiency in active ingredients or the presence of contaminants. Since the Food and Drug Administration (FDA) does not regulate nutritional supplements unless they cause a problem, this can be a good site for the millions of Americans taking these products.

In addition to what you can offer in the office you may also want to consider the partnerships you can foster through your clinic. Weight Watchers could hold meetings in your office after working hours. How about allowing the Lung Association's speaker to offer smoking cessation classes in your reception area during the Great American Smokeout? If you chose to partner with a dietician, you could host a healthy cooking or healthy shopping program once a month to help patients become better health consumers. There are many ideas that could work in the office setting; either during your day or after-hours. It will be up to you to determine what works best for you.

PARTNERSHIPS IN RURAL AREAS

There may be times when clinicians in rural areas find themselves somewhat isolated and with few resources seemingly available to them. Most land-grant universities have an extension service. The extension service from America's land-grant institutions is a part of the U.S. Department of Agriculture (USDA). Although the services cover a broad range of topics, including economic development, they also have health promotion and nutrition as focus areas to assist in improving health outcomes in rural communities. A description of those services can be found on the USDA website at: http://www.csrees.usda.gov/nea/food/food.cfm and these should be considered potential partners in your efforts to assist your patient-base in improving overall health goals.

Health fairs can also be organized in rural areas and the nearest farmer's market could serve as an education point for healthy shopping or healthy cooking classes. The extension agent would likely be helpful in setting up most programs to reach out to rural communities. In many cases, the state department of public health will have an office in the county and can have resources available. However, smaller branch offices of the public health department often have unfunded mandates for all sorts of programs, so resources could be stretched thin. It won't hurt to try. The next organization of interest is the state public health association. Often they have resources to help in rural outreach and may have members in your region. Since many county health workers, educators, and nutritionists belong to these organizations, partnering could be strength when you are few in number.

The other noteworthy potential partner in rural areas may be the nearest regional university. Some regional universities have a mission to serve underserved or rural populations, and they may have people employed in various departments who have special interest in helping small communities. Some states also have a division of rural community health and may have staff members who will help with health promotion, nutrition, and wellness programs in your region. In addition, for those rural areas near Native American Indian Reservations, tribal health agencies typically have a public health division that may be eager to work with you as well.

There is a lot to offer if you so choose. It may depend on your time availability, the staff you have, and resources in your particular area. Partnering with other professionals can be rewarding and is encouraged. That is the public health model. Setting up your office with a goal of moving patients toward positive health changes starts with deciding what you want to do and who you want to have involved. From there, within reason, the possibilities are unlimited!

Literature Cited

1. Smith PC, Schmidt SM, Allensworth-Davies D, et al. Primary care validation of a single-question alcohol screening test. *J Gen Intern Med*. 2009;24(7):783–788.

2. Stevens AM, Hennessy T, Baggett HC, et al. Methicillin-resistant Staphylococcus aureus carriage and risk factors for skin infections, Southwestern Alaska, USA. *Emerg Infect Dis*. 2010;16(5):797–803. http://wwwnc.cdc.gov/eid/article/16/5/09-0851.htm.

3. Cohen HA, Amir J, Matalon A, et al. Stethoscopes and otoscopes–a potential vector of infection? *Fam Pract*. 1997;14(6):446–449.

4. Puhl AA, Reinhart CJ, Puhl NJ, et al. An investigation of bacterial contamination on treatment table surfaces of chiropractors in private practice and attitudes and practices concerning table disinfection. *Am J Infect Control*. 2011;39(1):56–63.

5. United States Preventive Services Taskforce. *Guide to Clinical Preventive Services 2010–2011*. Rockville, MD: United States Preventive Services Taskforce. http://www.ahrq.gov/clinic/pocketgd1011/pocketgd1011.pdf. Accessed October 8, 2012.

6. SF-36 org.User's Manual for the SF-36 v2. http://www.sf-36.org. Accessed October 8, 2012.

7. About BMI for Children and Teens. Centers for Disease Control and Prevention. http://www.cdc.gov/healthyweight/assessing/bmi/childrens_bmi/about_childrens_bmi.html. Accessed October 8, 2012.

INDEX

Note: Page numbers followed by *f* indicate figures; those followed by *t* indicate tables.

Well-being/energy, assessment of, 53
Wellness assessment, 50–51. *See also* Preventive services;
    Worksite wellness; Health promotion
Wellness coaching
  development of
    challenges, 21
    confidence, 21
    goals, 22
    motivators, 21
    patient assessment, 18–21
    strategies, 22
    strengths, 21–22
    support, 22
    vision statement, 21
  versus health, 14
  principles of, 14–22
  theoretical basis of, 15
    attitude, 15
    techniques, 15–18
Wellness consultant/contractor, 147
Wellness Council of America (WECOA), 146

West Nile virus (WNV), 4
Whole egg, protein content in, 90*t*
Whole grain bread, protein content in, 90*t*
Worksite wellness (WW), 142–143
  clinicians in, 146–147
  generations of, 143–145
  health promotion, 142
  history of, 143–145
  successful programs, benchmarks of, 145–146
World Health Organization (WHO), 1, 90
World Wide Web, 35–36
  accuracy and coverage, 38
  authority, 36
  bias, 37–38
  currency, 36–37
  design, 38–39
WW. *See* Worksite wellness

Z

Zaleplon (Sonata), 131*t*
Zolpidem (Ambien), 131*t*